GERIATRIC CARE BY DESIGN:

A Clinician's Handbook to Meet the Needs of Older Adults through Environmental and Practice Redesign

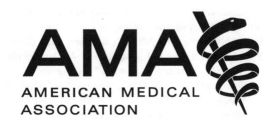

AMERICAN MEDICAL ASSOCIATION

Executive Vice President, Chief Executive Officer: James L. Madara, MD
Chief Operating Officer: Bernard L. Hengesbaugh
Editor-in-Chief: Audrey Chun, MD
Deputy Editors: Joanne G. Schwartzberg, MD and Cheryl Irmiter, PhD, LCSW, CADC
Project Manager: Kelly Towey, M.Ed
Manager, Book and Product Development and Production: Nancy Baker
Senior Developmental Editor: Lisa Chin-Johnson
Production Specialist: Mary Ann Albanese

ISBN 978-1-60359-658-9

TABLE OF CONTENTS

Structural Design

Evaluating Your Practice

Staffing and Human Resources

Coordination of Care

Care Coordination Models for Older Adults:

Other Issues Important to Care Coordination:

Role of the Family Caregiver

Health Literacy and Patient Self-Management

Culturally Effective Care

ABOUT THE CONTRIBUTORS

EDITOR IN CHIEF

Audrey Chun, MD
Martha Stewart Center for Living
Department of Geriatrics and Palliative Medicine
Mount Sinai School of Medicine, New York, New York

Dr Chun completed her residency in internal medicine at Baylor College of Medicine in Houston, Texas. She then finished her fellowship in geriatrics at the Mount Sinai School of Medicine, where she also served as chief fellow. As a recipient of a Health Professions Health Resources and Services Administration (HRSA)–funded Geriatric Academic Career Award (GACA), she is able to pursue her clinical interests, which include geriatric assessment, medical education, and delivery of care models in the outpatient setting. She is active in the educational programs of geriatrics and palliative care and regularly participates in the education of medical students, residents, geriatrics fellows, and colleagues at her home institution and nationally. She has been featured in the Frontline documentary "Living Old" and has participated in numerous panel discussions on aging in America and its implications. She was also recently awarded a Practice Change Fellowship funded through the Hartford Foundation and Atlantic Philanthropies that will focus on improving care for older adults. Currently, she is the director of the Martha Stewart Center for Living at the Mount Sinai Medical Center and the director of clinical services in the Department of Geriatrics and Palliative Medicine.

DEPUTY EDITORS

Joanne G. Schwartzberg, MD
Aging and Community Health
American Medical Association, Chicago, Illinois

Dr Schwartzberg is director of aging and community health at the American Medical Association. She received her BA from Harvard and MD from Northwestern and is a clinical assistant professor of preventive medicine and community health at the University of Illinois at Chicago College of Medicine. Dr Schwartzberg is a past president of the Institute of Medicine of Chicago, the Illinois Geriatrics Society, and the American Academy of Home Care Physicians.

In 1988 she received the Physician of the Year Award from the National Association for Home Care. In 1992 she received the Physician of the Year Award from the American Academy of Home Care Physicians. In 1995 she served as cochair of the Illinois delegation to the White House Conference on Aging, Caucus on Health and Social Services. She was a presidential appointee to the Advisory Committee of the 2005 White House Conference on Aging. She is a member of the Safe Medication Use Expert Committee for the United States Pharmacopeia (USP). She currently directs a variety of AMA national initiatives at the undergraduate, graduate, and postgraduate level to develop physician competency in caring for the aging patient.

Dr Schwartzberg is the 2001 recipient of the Henry P. Russe, MD "Citation for Exemplary Compassion in Healthcare" awarded by the Institute of Medicine of Chicago and the Rush-Presbyterian-St Luke's Medical Center.

Cheryl Irmiter, PhD, LCSW, CADC
Aging and Community Health
American Medical Association, Chicago, Illinois

Dr Irmiter is a PhD clinical social worker. She is a senior scientist for the American Medical Association in the Division of Medicine and Public Health Division, and the Department of Aging and Community Health. She is an adjunct faculty member of Loyola University Chicago and has taught human behavior and research courses at the University of Chicago Social Service Administration Program and Northwestern University's Feinberg School of Medicine. Before her work at the AMA, she was a research fellow at the University of Michigan, Department of Psychiatry, Mental Health Services Outcomes and Translations Section, and the Ann Arbor Veterans Health Administration.

Dr Irmiter has more than 14 years of direct clinical care experience working with adults and older adults in community medical and psychiatric health care. She has had a significant number of publications and presentations throughout her career and has been nominated for and received various awards recognizing her scholarship and ability to bridge clinical practice and research for the underserved.

ADVISORY EDITOR

Rosanne M. Leipzig, MD, PhD
Department of Geriatric and Palliative Medicine
Mount Sinai School of Medicine, New York, New York

Rosanne M. Leipzig, MD, PhD, is the Gerald and Mary Ellen Ritter Professor (tenured) and the Vice Chair for Education of the Brookdale Department of Geriatrics and Adult Development at the Mount Sinai School of Medicine in New York. Dr. Leipzig graduated from the University of Rochester, received her MD and PhD (Human Genetics) at the University of Michigan Medical Center, completed her internal medicine residency at the University of Rochester and a Fellowship in Clinical Pharmacology at New York Hospital/Cornell University Medical Center, and has been recognized with numerous national awards for excellence in medical education and geriatrics. Dr Leipzig's research and publications highlight evidence-based treatment for older adults, the use of restraints in hospitalized elderly, and models for teaching geriatrics, chronic care, and evidence-based medicine. She is a member of the Board of Directors for the American Board of Internal Medicine and serves on the United States Preventive Services Task Force.

SECTION EDITORS

Heidi Auerbach, MD
Section of Geriatrics
Boston University Medical Center, Boston, Massachusetts

Dr Auerbach completed her residency in primary care internal medicine at the Johns Hopkins Bayview Medical Center in Baltimore, Maryland, and then served for 1 year as chief resident. She completed a 2-year fellowship in geriatric medicine and gerontology at the Johns Hopkins School of Medicine. She has been medical director of Boston Medical Center's Geriatric Ambulatory Practice since its inception in 1997 and continues to work on performance improvement and clinical design changes as the practice evolves. She has also been actively involved with the development of electronic health record geriatric screening forms, previously funded through her institution's Comprehensive Geriatric Education Project grant from the Donald W. Reynolds Foundation. She is a faculty member of Boston University's Center of Excellence Scholars Program and the Chief Resident Immersion Training Program in the Care of Older Adults, both currently supported by the John A. Hartford Foundation. She is active in multiple educational endeavors for the Section of Geriatrics, including ongoing teaching of medical students and geriatric medicine fellows in the ambulatory setting.

Rosemary Bakker, MS
Division of Geriatrics
National Academy for Psychosocial Health on Aging
Weill Cornell Medical College, New York, New York

Rosemary Bakker is a gerontologist and a certified interior designer and is on academic staff at Weill Cornell Medical College. During the last 15 years, Ms Bakker has assumed a national and local leadership role in promoting the role of the environment to optimize the health, function, and well-being of older adults. She has conducted safety assessments in a variety of environments, including single-family homes, senior housing, and health care facilities.

Ms Bakker was one of three primary investigators covered under a 4-year physician education grant awarded by the Donald W. Reynolds Foundation to the Weill Cornell Geriatric Division for her online animated course for health professionals, Environmental Geriatrics. Ms Bakker was awarded a 3-year Investigator-Initiated Research Grant from the Alzheimer's Association for her current project, ThisCaringHome.org, a multimedia Web site on best practices in home safety and dementia care.

Ms Bakker has authored two books on design, aging, and wellness, including AARP's *Guide to Revitalizing Your Home* (2010) (and is a one of Dr Oz's 100 Expert Advisors). She has made numerous presentations to diverse audiences, including health care professionals, interior designers, housing experts, Fortune

500 corporations, Centers for Disease Control and Prevention, the Museum of Modern Art, the Alzheimer's Association, and the United Nations.

Eileen Callahan, MD
Department of Geriatrics and Palliative Medicine
Mount Sinai School of Medicine, New York, New York

Dr Callahan is board certified in internal medicine, geriatric medicine, and palliative medicine. On completion of her geriatric medicine fellowship at Mount Sinai Medical Center, Dr Callahan joined the Mount Sinai faculty, where she is currently associate professor in the Brookdale Department of Geriatrics and Palliative Medicine and the Department of Internal Medicine. From 1997 to 2006, her primary clinical and educational venue was the Acute Care for the Elderly (ACE) Unit, where as medical director Dr Callahan established a setting that provides quality hospital care for geriatric patients and served as a teaching site for the education of students of all disciplines, including medicine, nursing, social work, and physical therapy. Her work is now focused at the Coffey Geriatrics Ambulatory Care Practice at the Martha Stewart Center for Living, where she is an administrative firm chief and provides consultative and primary care to the community elderly and teaches the fellows in geriatric medicine. She has established a caregiver's program to provide education and support for caregivers of patients with dementia.

Elizabeth Eckstrom, MD, MPH
Division of General Internal Medicine and Geriatrics
Oregon Health & Science University, Portland, Oregon

Dr Eckstrom is associate professor and director of geriatrics at Oregon Health & Science University (OHSU) in Portland. She received her MD degree from the University of Wisconsin, then headed west to complete residency and fellowship at OHSU, as well as an MPH through the University of Washington. She practices both primary care and consultative geriatrics, and specializes in promoting an active lifestyle in older adults and issues relevant to healthy aging in women. Her research has focused on physical activity in older adults and studying the effectiveness of training primary care faculty to improve their care of older adults. She teaches medical students and internal medicine residents, and works with inpatient teams to improve quality of care for older hospitalized patients throughout the institution. She is principal investigator for the Oregon Geriatric Education Center, working with OHSU's Schools of Nursing, Dentistry, and Pharmacy; PSU's Institute on Aging; and OSU's gerontology program to find solutions to challenges facing older adults.

Alex Federman, MD, MPH
Division of General Internal Medicine
Mount Sinai School of Medicine, New York, New York

Dr Federman is an assistant professor of medicine in the Division of General Internal Medicine at Mount Sinai School of Medicine, where he joined the faculty in September 2002. Dr Federman was awarded a Robert Wood Johnson

Generalist Physician Faculty Scholarship in 2004 and a Paul B. Beeson Career Development Award in Aging Research from the National Institute on Aging in 2006. Dr Federman is an aging-related health services and behavioral health researcher, with a focus on health literacy and cognition. His work is conducted in the context of health insurance issues for older adults, physician-patient communication about medication and health care costs, generic medication use by the elderly, and health care reform. In addition to his research activities, Dr Federman is a deputy editor at the *Journal of General Internal Medicine*. He also co-directs the research training fellowship in general internal medicine at Mount Sinai Hospital, supervises medical residents, and provides outpatient primary care to a panel of patients from the socioeconomically diverse populations of Central and East Harlem and the South Bronx in New York.

Won Lee, MD
Boston University Medical Center, Boston, Massachusetts

Dr Lee completed her residency in internal medicine at Tufts Medical Center and her geriatric medicine fellowship at Boston Medical Center, both in Boston. As a clinician educator, she is focused on the education and training of medical students and residents while practicing in the Boston Medical Center's Geriatric Ambulatory Practice, in the historic and very active Home Care Program, and on the Geriatrics Inpatient Service. Her clinical interests include group patient visits and medical education. She has been selected to participate in the Harvard Macy Institute 2011 Program for Educators in Health Professions.

Matthew McNabney, MD
Division of Geriatric Medicine and Gerontology
Johns Hopkins School of Medicine, Baltimore, Maryland

Dr McNabney graduated from the University of Missouri–Kansas City School of Medicine and completed his residency in internal medicine at Northwestern University and his fellowship in geriatric medicine at UCLA. He is currently the fellowship program director in geriatric medicine at Johns Hopkins, as well as the medical director of Hopkins ElderPlus (a Program of All-Inclusive Care for the Elderly, or PACE). Dr McNabney is vice chair of the Clinical Practice and Models of Care Committee of the American Geriatrics Society, which is responsible for establishing and evaluating practice guidelines for the care of older adults. He also serves on the Primary Care Committee and is chairman of the Research Committee of the National PACE Association. He has written several peer-reviewed articles in the area of long-term care.

Arun S. Rao, MD
Assistant Program Director, Geriatric Medicine Fellowship Program
Medical Director, Gruss-Lipper House Call Program
Weill Cornell Medical College, New York, New York

Dr Rao completed his undergraduate medical education at UMDNJ–Robert Wood Johnson Medical School. He did his internship and residency in internal medicine there as well and a fellowship in geriatric medicine at the University of

Michigan Medical School in Ann Arbor. On completing his fellowship, he joined the faculty in the Division of Geriatrics and Gerontology at Weill Cornell Medical College in 2002. He currently serves as the assistant program director for the Geriatric Medicine Fellowship Program at Cornell and also as the medical director of the Gruss-Lipper House Call Program of Weill Cornell Medical College. The recipient of two Geriatric Academic Career Awards, Dr Rao has a strong interest in ethnicity and aging as well as providing training in teaching skills to geriatric medicine fellows. He has completed coursework at the Harvard Macy Institute's Program for Physician Educators and the Stanford University Geriatric Education Center's Faculty Development Program in Health Literacy and Ethnogeriatrics. Dr Rao currently serves on the Ethnogeriatrics Committee of the American Geriatrics Society and on the Task Force on Minority Issues for the Health Sciences Section of the Gerontological Society of America.

PROJECT MANAGER

Kelly Towey, MEd
Communications Consultant
AMA Aging and Community Health

CONTRIBUTING AUTHORS:

Mahnaz Ahmad, MD, MS
Geriatric Medicine
Legacy Clinic Good Samaritan
Portland, Oregon

John R. Anderson, MD
Division of Geriatric Medicine
Mt Auburn Hospital
Cambridge, Massachusetts

Alicia I. Arbaje, MD, MPH
Division of Geriatric Medicine and Gerontology
Johns Hopkins University

Heidi Auerbach, MD
Section of Geriatrics
Boston University Medical Center
Boston, Massachusetts

Kevin T. Bain, PharmD, MPH, BCPS, CGP, CPH, FASCP, CCA
excelleRx, Inc, an Omnicare Company
Philadelphia, Pennsylvania

Rosemary Bakker, MS
Division of Geriatrics
National Academy for Psychosocial Health on Aging
Weill Cornell Medical College
New York, New York

John M. Bruza, MD
Division of Geriatric Medicine
University of Pennsylvania Health System
Philadelphia, Pennsylvania

Arline Bohannon, MD
VCU Health System
Richmond, Virginia

Chad Boult, MD, MPH, MBA
Roger C. Lipitz Center for Integrated Health Care
Johns Hopkins Bloomberg School of Public Health
Baltimore, Maryland

John M. Bruza, MD
Division of Geriatric Medicine
Penn Presbyterian Medical Center
University of Pennsylvania Health System

Kristy Butler, PharmD, BCPS
Division of General Internal Medicine & Geriatrics
Oregon Health and Science University
Portland, Oregon

Eileen H. Callahan, MD
Mount Sinai School of Medicine
New York, New York

Lisa Caruso, MD, MPH
Section of Geriatrics
Boston University Medical Center
Boston Massachusetts

Grace I. Chen, MD
Division of Geriatrics
David Geffen School of Medicine at UCLA
Los Angeles, California

Audrey Chun, MD
Martha Stewart Center for Living
Department of Geriatric and Palliative Medicine
Mount Sinai School of Medicine
New York, New York

Connie L. Davis, GNP, BC
Connie L. Davis Health Services Ltd
Chilliwack, British Columbia, Canada

Melinda Davis, MA, PhD candidate
Oregon Rural Practice-Based Research Network
Oregon Health & Science University
Portland, Oregon

Elizabeth Eckstrom, MD, MPH
Division of General Internal Medicine and Geriatrics
Oregon Health & Science University
Portland, Oregon

Lyle J. (LJ) Fagnan, MD
Oregon Rural Practice-based Research Network
Oregon Health & Science University
Portland, Oregon

Alex Federman, MD, MPH
Division of General Internal Medicine
Mount Sinai School of Medicine
New York, New York

Ian Ferrari, PharmD candidate 2010
Pacific University Oregon School of Pharmacy
Hillsboro, Oregon

Elizabeth G. Fine, LCSW
Mount Sinai School of Medicine
New York, New York

Angela Gentili, MD
Geriatrics Fellowship Program
VCU Health System and McGuire VA Medical Center
Richmond, Virginia

Monica Goubaud, MA, CCRP
Oregon Rural Practice-Based Research Network
Oregon Health & Science University
Portland, Oregon

Steven M. Handler, MD, PhD, CMD
University of Pittsburgh School of Medicine
Department of Biomedical Informatics and Division of Geriatric Medicine
Geriatric Research Education and Clinical Center (GRECC)
Veterans Affairs Pittsburgh Healthcare System
Pittsburgh, Pennsylvania

James Judge, MD
Evercare Connecticut
University of Connecticut School of Medicine
Farmington, Connecticut

Margaret Kelly, BS, RN
Section of Geriatrics
Boston University Medical Center
Boston, Massachusetts

Ilona Kopits, MD, MPH
Boston University Geriatrics Services
Boston Medical Center
PACE Upham's Corner Community Health Center
Boston, Massachusetts

Brandon Koretz, MD
Division of Geriatric Medicine
David Geffen School of Medicine at UCLA
Los Angeles, California

Seema Limaye, MD
Section of Geriatrics and Palliative Medicine
University of Chicago
Chicago, Illinois

Won Lee, MD
Section of Geriatrics
Boston University Medical Center
Boston, Massachusetts

Allison Lindauer, FNP, GNP
Division of General Internal Medicine and Geriatrics
Oregon Health & Science University
Portland, Oregon

Jeffrey Mariano, MD
Department of Geriatrics/Palliative/Continuing Care
Kaiser Permanente Southern California
Los Angeles, California

Ann McDonough, MS, RN
Geriatric Ambulatory Practice
Boston Medical Center
Boston, Massachusetts

Matthew McNabney, MD
Division of Geriatric Medicine and Gerontology
Hopkins ElderPlus
Johns Hopkins University
Baltimore, Maryland

David Mehr, MD, MS
MU Family and Community Medicine
University of Missouri School of Medicine

Paul Mulhausen, MD MHS
Division of General Internal Medicine
University of Iowa Carver College of Medicine
Iowa City, Iowa

Margaret B. Neal, PhD
Institute on Aging
School of Community Health, College of Urban and Public Affairs
Portland State University
Portland, Oregon

Tracy Novak, MHS
The Roger C. Lipitz Center for Integrated Health Care
Department of Health Policy and Management
Johns Hopkins Bloomberg School of Public Health
Baltimore, Maryland

Daniel Oates, MD, MSc
Boston University School of Medicine
Boston Medical Center
Boston, Massachusetts

Arun S. Rao, MD
Geriatric Medicine Fellowship Program
Gruss-Lipper House Call Program
Weill Cornell Medical College
New York, New York

David B. Reuben, MD
Division of Geriatric Medicine
Multicampus Program in Geriatric Medicine and Gerontology
David Geffen School of Medicine at UCLA
Los Angeles, California

Sonja Rosen, MD
Department of Internal Medicine
Division of Geriatric Medicine
UCLA David Geffen School of Medicine
Los Angeles, California

Debbi Shackelford
Patient Access Services Specialist
Oregon Health & Science University
Portland, Oregon

Beata Skudlarska, MD, CMD
Bridgeport Hospital Center for Geriatrics
Yale New Haven Health System
Yale School of Medicine
New Haven, Connecticut

Robin Telerant, MD
Oregon Health & Science University
Portland, Oregon

Dante Tipiani, MSW
Department of Geriatric Psychiatry
Mount Sinai Medical Center
New York, New York

John H. Wasson, MD
Dartmouth Medical School
Hanover, New Hampshire

Diana L. White, PhD
Institute on Aging
School of Community Health, College of Urban and Public Affairs
Portland State University
Portland, Oregon

Michael S. Wolf, PhD, MPH
Division of General Internal Medicine
Feinberg School of Medicine
Northwestern University
Chicago, Illinois

REVIEWERS:

Lynda A. Anderson, PhD

Alejandro Aparicio, MD, FACP

John Burton, MD

Barry D. Dickinson, PhD

George Drach, MD

Doug Fedorchak

Susan A. Forbes, CID, ASID, DLF, IDEC

Margaret Gadon, MD, MPH

Lorna Lynn, MD

Doriane Miller, MD

Marie Mindeman, RHIT

James S. Powers, MD

Alice Reed

David B. Reuben, MD

Donna Rosenstiel, LCSW

Karen Sauvigne, MA

Patricia Sokol, RN, JD

Geoffrey B. Walton, MHA

James Webster, MD, MS, MACP

Nancy Whitelaw, PhD

PREFACE

It is an honor and a privilege to write the preface to this first edition of *Geriatric Care by Design*. Conceived as a practical online resource, the goal of this e-book is to advance the physician and older-patient relationship by providing information on office design strategies that optimize the health care setting. We recognize that each of these sections and some of the chapters could and do have entire books dedicated to the subject. However, we also know that busy clinicians need concise information with links to resources for additional investigation, as needed.

My own experience with practice redesign highlights the lack of cohesive resources in considering practice design for older adults. My colleagues and I recognized the need to address practice management from a geriatric perspective as we planned a move from one space to another. What type of examination table is best for older adults? How large should the rooms be? How many rooms do we need? How can we have large enough examination rooms *and* the number of rooms necessary to facilitate flow? Through these questions, it became clear that attention to the physical space was only one aspect of the necessary redesign. In addition to negotiating space, furniture, and physical access, there were a number of other areas that needed to be adapted or implemented to improve patient care. The physical redesign highlighted additional opportunities to promote related but distinct areas of patient care ranging from scheduling and staff development to visit flow and care coordination.

Older adults require specific design considerations that could be incorporated into medical practices for all patients. For example, because of age-related eye changes that include decreased pupillary size and adaptation, patient materials should be printed with high-contrast colors (black and white) and paper that minimizes glare (matte instead of glossy). Most of us were never trained in some of these changes that occur with aging, much less how to translate them into daily practice to facilitate care.

Because there are few resources that address both physical and systems design for older adults, this e-book aims to be a practical guide on how to improve the quality of care for older patients by design that meets the needs of physicians, patients, and office staff. Through the experiences of experts who struggle daily with the universal challenges of finite space, resources, and staffing, this book contains pragmatic plans and templates for making changes both big and small. It is formatted to fit the lives of busy practitioners through bulleted points and easy-to-use checklists, tables, and links to resources. We fully expect that any practice caring for older adults can implement at least some of these recommendations within the context of their own practice, whether it is primary or specialty care.

I also want to take this opportunity to thank those who made this book possible. The mentorship of Dr. Rosanne Leipzig along with the vision of our deputy editors, Cheryl Irmiter, PhD and Dr. Joanne Schwartzberg, moved this project from idea to reality. Kelly Towey, our project manager, kept everything organized and on track. Our section editors and authors have committed countless hours and ideas to the formation of this project. Their enthusiasm and experiences are the heart of this handbook.

While the process of practice improvement is never-ending, we hope this book provides the basics for considering the ambulatory practice as a conduit for excellent patient care, especially for older adults.

Audrey Chun, MD Editor-in-Chief

CHAPTER ONE

Environmental Design

Rosemary Bakker, MS

MRS JOHNSON'S EXPERIENCE

This is Mrs Johnson's first visit to your office. Leaving the parking lot, she struggles to lift her walker over the curb and onto the sidewalk. Approaching the clinic's entrance, she notices four steps she cannot climb; inquiries to passersby reveal that there is a delivery ramp in the back. Inside the building, she wanders the corridors before finding a sign directing her to the right elevator. As she enters your office, she turns her hearing aid up high but still has difficulty understanding the receptionist, who is seated behind a glass partition. When called for her appointment, she ambulates with a cautious gait, as the shiny flooring appears slick to her from reflected overhead lighting. Once in the examination room, she is embarrassed to ask for help getting on and off the high examination table. When her appointment is finished, a staff member accompanies her down a long, steep hallway to an exit with only one step. Though the staff helps place her walker on ground level, there are no handrails to hold for support. She feels vulnerable and unsafe and knows she cannot come again without help.

The case is exaggerated to include multiple barriers in the designed environment that cause functional limitations, but every element was taken from a physician's office I have visited.

INTRODUCTION

Because of chronic conditions that accrue with advancing age, both age-related conditions such as hearing loss and disease conditions such as arthritis or macular degeneration, older adults encounter an increasing array of environmental barriers that compromise function. When decreased functioning or injury occurs, however, the common misperception is that the problems are due solely to age-related functional decline, rather than to the dynamic interface between the older user's capabilities and the designed environment. In addition, changing demographics indicate that the problems of functional decline and environmental access go beyond advancing age; one in five Americans is now reported to have a disability.[1] The American with Disabilities Act (ADA) legally mandates that health care facilities, including clinics and private offices, meet the environmental needs of patients with disabilities, regardless of age. Though the geriatric population benefits from accessibility requirements, there are additional design considerations essential for this cohort. This chapter will list key code requirements along with age-friendly design recommendations that can serve as a planning guide for creating a health care environment in which patients with a range of conditions can function more independently and safely.

OPPORTUNITIES

➤ Increase the number of patients who can easily access the office, from teenagers on crutches to centenarians in wheelchairs. Providing access also includes consideration for family members and caregivers, vital components of the geriatric health care team.

➤ Reduce fall risk and liability, as falls among older adults in which the designed environment is a contributing factor are common.

➤ Improve patient function, as a well-designed, age-friendly environment can increase visual, auditory, cognitive, and physical skills, which enhances patient participation and self-esteem.

➤ Improve staff efficiency and reduce stress of patient care through increased patient function.

➤ Reduce legal liability through compliance with both ADA and Health Insurance Portability and Accountability Act (HIPAA) requirements.

> ➤ The ADA requires that all health care buildings, including private offices, comply with the design and construction standards contained in the Americans with Disability Act Accessibility Guidelines (ADAAG). These guidelines cover new construction, additions, or renovation of existing office spaces, depending on reasonable costs.

> ➤ Improve HIPAA privacy through appropriate space planning and acoustical control.

➤ Begin large or small. Though cost can be a barrier to major structural renovations, many age-friendly changes can be made without great expense:

    ➤ Higher light levels to enhance vision and mobility

    ➤ Ramp added for patients and visitors with mobility impairments

    ➤ Enhanced acoustical control to facilitate communication

    ➤ Appropriate seating and examination tables for safer transfers

    ➤ Safer flooring, including low-pile carpeting, matte finishes on wood, linoleum, or vinyl, and low thresholds.

CHALLENGES

➤ Cost can be an issue, depending on the scope of the project and available funds. For new construction, the marginal cost for constructing an age-friendly environment is relatively small (estimated at 1% to 5%). For renovation, cost can vary dramatically and create obstacles, depending on the structural changes needed.

➤ Space and legal limitations include inadequate floor space for larger examination rooms and bathrooms, an elevator, ramp, or lift, and leases that contain limits on renovations.

➤ Time constraints and patient inconvenience (eg, noise, construction dust) may be limiting factors.

SOLUTIONS

When planning or renovating a health care facility, clinic, or office (or even a private home), the following three strategies, presented in Tables 1-1, 1-2, and 1-3, are designed to be used in developing an age-friendly health care environment. They provide information on geriatric design considerations in a convenient format and can be used as a practical tool when working with administrators, architects, designers, and other health care professionals.

1. Review and plan by *design implications of age and disease-related changes*

2. Review and plan by *area and functional needs*

3. Review and plan *by design element*

Together, the tables provide a broad overview; however, as readers may prefer to consider design issues primarily from one point of view, some information is purposely included in more than one table.

TABLE 1-1 Design Implications of Age- and Disease-Related Changes
The health care environment can cause unnecessary discomfort, or even disability, if the functional needs of older patients are not accommodated in the office design. Age-friendly design, on the other hand, contributes to safety, function, and well-being of all patients.

Vision	Hearing
➤ Heightened sensitivity to glare (especially on flooring surfaces, impeding safe movement)	➤ Inability to hear conversations in environments with background noise
➤ Slow adaptation to changes in light level	➤ Loss of hearing in high-frequency range (eg, female speech)
➤ Reduced depth perception (especially for flooring and stairs)	➤ Inability to hear certain words
➤ Reduced field of vision	➤ Sensitivity to loud sounds
➤ Reduced visual acuity	➤ Hearing aids not always effective

Strength and Mobility	Cognitive Function
➤ Changes in gait and balance, loss of muscle strength, and abnormalities in the central nervous and musculoskeletal systems decrease capacity for: ➤ Stair climbing, especially without handrails ➤ Walking long distances, especially if occasional seating is not provided ➤ Rising from low seating or examination tables ➤ Rising from toilets without grab bars ➤ Walking or wheeling over raised door sills	➤ Wayfinding issues, even in smaller offices ➤ Problems with visual/spatial perception if foreground/background are not color-contrasted (eg, edges of steps) ➤ Perceptual distortion caused by highly patterned flooring, seating, or wall covering and by reflective surfaces, including mirrors and bare windows ➤ Hypersensitivity and inability to focus due to excessive background noise ➤ Inability to understand instructions or communication spoken quickly in complex sentences

TABLE 1-2 Functional Solutions by Area

This table reviews common problems in each *area* of the office or facility and provides corresponding solutions. Key ADAAG requirements are also included.

PARKING AREAS AND WALKWAYS	
Problems	**Solutions**
➤ Uneven walking surfaces, eg, gravel, potholes	➤ Paved level surfaces and gently sloped walkways
	➤ *Vigilant* repair of holes and other surface irregularities
➤ High curbs	➤ Curb cutouts
	➤ Curbs and other variations in walking surface highlighted with bright contrasting color (eg, yellow)
➤ Low light levels, especially at dusk	➤ Ample glare-free lighting in garages and along walkways at dusk
➤ Long walking distances	➤ Ample reserved parking near offices and benches along walkways

STAIRS—OUTDOORS AND INDOORS	
Problems	**Solutions**
➤ Lack of alternatives to stairs	➤ Stair alternatives
	➤ Ramp (1:12 maximum incline)
	➤ Wheelchair lift
	➤ Stair glider chair
	➤ Elevator (if space and budget allow)
➤ Unsafe stairs	➤ Stairs with safety features
➤ No or only one handrail (especially for people with one-sided weakness)	➤ Handrails on both sides of stairs (even for one step), and extended beyond step at top and bottom for gait stabilization
➤ Edges of steps not easily seen	➤ Edges of steps highlighted with 2-inch strip of bright contrasting color (eg, yellow)
➤ Patterned carpet on stairs	➤ Nonpatterned stair carpet
➤ Low light levels	➤ Adequate glare-free lighting

(continued)

TABLE 1-2 *(continued)*

ENTRANCE

Problems	Solutions
➤ Entrance difficult to find	➤ Clearly designated entryway (eg, large address plaque, colorful awning)
	➤ Sufficient lighting for overcast days and dusk
➤ Lack of weather protection	➤ Roof overhang or awning over entryway
➤ Inadequate maneuvering space at doorway for patients in wheelchairs	➤ Approximately 5 × 5 ft of floor space and adequate clearance on latch side of door
➤ Door difficult to open for patients using mobility devices or those with limited strength	➤ Automatic door or lightweight door with lever handle (requiring no more than 5 lbs of force to operate)
➤ Raised thresholds impede mobility for patients with:	➤ Entrance without threshold or reduced threshold (see Flooring section)
➤ mobility device	➤ Contrasting color on raised threshold to improve visibility
➤ walking impairments	
➤ visual/spatial impairments	
➤ Temporarily impaired vision inside entrance due to change in light level (outside/inside)	➤ Brighter lighting inside door to accommodate older patients' slow adjustment to light level change
➤ Slippery flooring	➤ Provision for absorbent flooring for rain or snow

HALLWAYS

Problems	Solutions
➤ No handrails or handrails not easily graspable	➤ Handrails on both sides, easily graspable (eg, round or oval, 1¼- to 1½-in diameter)
➤ Disabling glare on flooring	➤ Matte floor finish or low-pile carpeting
➤ Obstructed pathway (eg, carts or storage)	➤ Sufficient storage space to clear pathways

➤ Narrow hallways	➤ Wider hallways to accommodate
	➤ traffic flow
	➤ wheelchair turns into bathrooms/ offices
	➤ patients with caregivers

RECEPTION AND WAITING AREA: SAFE MOBILITY AND ACCESS

Problems	Solutions
➤ Inaccessible reception desk	➤ Wheelchair-accessible countertop area 36 in wide (minimum) by 30 in high
➤ Unsafe flooring (eg slippery finishes, area carpets, dark or highly patterned carpeting)	➤ Matte floor finishes or low-pile carpeting to improve mobility
	➤ Light to medium floor colors
	➤ No patterns, or simple patterns with low color contrast to improve perception
➤ Inadequate space for mobility device plus caregiver	➤ 5 × 5-ft turning area for wheelchairs and walkers and space to maneuver mobility aides in seating areas
➤ Low tables, especially glass	➤ Safer tables that are not easily tripped over or bumped into, including nonglass tables and tables with rounded edges

RECEPTION AND WAITING AREA: COMMUNICATION

Problems	Solutions
➤ HIPAA noncompliance and lack of privacy	➤ Space for private consultation
➤ Background noise	➤ Sound-absorbing materials (eg, carpeting, drapes, acoustical wall panels and ceiling tile)
	➤ Eliminated/reduced volume: public address system, television, radio, and telephone
	➤ Assistive listening devices with headset and microphone available for patient use
➤ Staff located behind glass partition without amplification system	➤ Intercom system

(continued)

TABLE 1-2 *(continued)*

RECEPTION AND WAITING AREA: TRANSFERRING

Problems	Solutions
➤ Lack of functional seating that meets needs of multiple users	➤ Variety of seating choices for comfort and ease of transferring (see Seating section)
➤ Lack of supportive seat cushions (eg, soft or worn out seating that provides inadequate support when seated or transferring)	➤ Firm or medium-firm cushions specified and replaced as needed

BATHROOM: ACCESS AND SAFE MOBILITY

Problems	Solutions
➤ Narrow, inaccessible doorway for patients using scooter or wheelchair	➤ Wider doorway
➤ High threshold difficult to walk or wheel over; increases fall risk for patient with mobility or visual/spatial impairments	➤ No threshold or low-threshold ➤ Threshold in contrasting color for better visibility
➤ Limited floor space	➤ Enlarged space with 5 × 5-ft area for turning ➤ Adequate toilet transfer space: ADA specifications for front, diagonal, and side transfers are 48 × 66, 48 × 56, and 60 × 56 in, respectively
➤ Inaccessible sink for wheelchair users	➤ Sink with open space below ➤ Soap/towel dispenser reachable from sitting position
➤ Faucet knobs unusable by patients with weakened grip	➤ Automatic on/off faucet with controlled water temperature, or lever faucets
➤ Slippery flooring	➤ Matte floor finishes

BATHROOM: EMERGENCY COMMUNICATION AND ACCESS

Problems	Solutions
➤ Lack of accessible emergency call system (for patients who need help but may be unwilling to shout for assistance or may not be heard from a distance)	➤ Call system with large, color-contrasted text and pull cord color that contrasts with wall color (eg, red cord against white wall)

➤ Door swings into bathroom; patient may fall and block opening of door	➤ Door installed on two-way (double action) hinges that swing both ways for emergency access
➤ Locked door that cannot be opened from outside	➤ Bathroom lock operable from both inside and outside bathroom

BATHROOM: TOILET USAGE

Problems	Solutions
➤ Standard height toilet (14–16 in) difficult to rise from	➤ ADA-compliant height toilet (17–19 in), with elongated bowl for easier wheelchair transfers
➤ Lack of grab bars	➤ ADA-complaint grab bars ➤ Hinged grab bars on side for patients who benefit from pressing down to rise

➤ Lack of color contrast	➤ Color contrast for:
	
	  ➤ Grab bar to wall
	
	  ➤ Toilet seat to floor
	
	  ➤ Tinted toilet water to improve male patient aim

BATHROOM: WAYFINDING, VISUAL AND COGNITIVE ISSUES

Problems	Solutions
➤ Confusion or getting lost finding bathroom	➤ Signage on door with large, color-contrasted text and symbol (eg, "Bathroom" with toilet icon) ➤ Different door color than adjacent doors
➤ Getting lost exiting bathroom	➤ Signage viewable by patient exiting bathroom, directing patient to waiting area or physician's office

EXAMINATION ROOM/PHYSICIAN'S OFFICE: SAFE MOBILITY AND ACCESS

Problems	Solutions
➤ Narrow doorways	➤ Wheelchair-accessible doorways, with minimum clear opening of 32 in
➤ Inadequate floor space	➤ Larger room, including 5 × 5-ft turning area for mobility device and room for caregiver

(continued)

TABLE 1-2 *(continued)*

EXAMINATION ROOM/PHYSICIAN'S OFFICE: COMMUNICATION	
Problems	**Solutions**
➤ Sound transmission ➤ HIPAA noncompliance and lack of privacy	➤ Use of sound-absorbing materials and avoidance of materials that transmit sound (eg, glass inset in office door)
➤ Difficulty with patient communication	➤ Assistive listening device with headset and microphone

EXAMINATION ROOM/PHYSICIAN'S OFFICE: SEATING AND TRANSFERRING	
Problems	**Solutions**
➤ Fixed-height examination table	➤ Height-adjustable examination table; lowers to allow access for mobility impaired
➤ Inadequate chair design	➤ Seating with comfortable back, seat, and side arms

TABLE 1-3 Functional Solutions by Design Element

This table reviews how particular *design elements* should be treated for the benefit of older patients.

LIGHTING AND COLOR
Recommendations

Lighting

➤ Higher, glare-free light levels; all light sources shaded, including windows and light bulbs

➤ Consistent lighting from one area to next, including from outside to inside building

➤ Avoid exclusive reliance on ceiling and soffit lighting

➤ Task lighting for patient activities, especially for reading and completing forms

➤ Automatic sensor lighting as appropriate

Color

➤ Light to medium colors

   ➤ Effective light reflectance to improve visibility

   ➤ Dark colors perceived as black to aging eyes

➤ Warm rich colors (yellows, blue/greens) for a less institutional ambiance

Color Contrasting

➤ Define foreground/background

  ➤ Chair seat/floor

  ➤ Door trim/door

  ➤ Door handle/door

  ➤ Wall/floor intersection

  ➤ Grab bars/wall

  ➤ Faucets/sink

  ➤ Emergency pull cord/wall

Color/Pattern

➤ Use different color for stairs than for adjacent flooring

➤ Avoid strong dark/light flooring contrasts (eg, patients with perception problems may see dark borders as holes or depressions)

➤ Avoid *any* strong pattern

SIGNAGE AND WAYFINDING

Recommendations

➤ Consistent signage with large color-contrasted text and icon, as appropriate (eg, "Bathroom" with toilet icon)

➤ Signage at appropriate intervals to help prevent persons with cognitive impairment from getting lost

➤ Nonglare finishes

➤ Color or landmark to identify important area (eg, bright wall color and/or artwork)

ACOUSTICS AND SOUND CONTROL

Recommendations

➤ Sound-absorbing materials (eg, carpeting, window treatment, cubicle curtains, acoustical wall panels, and ceiling tile)

➤ Appropriate space planning and building material specification for reduced sound transmission

➤ Intercom system for effective communication when glass partition is used

➤ Eliminated/reduced volume: public address system, television, radio, and telephone

➤ Assistive listening devices with headset and microphone available for patient use

(continued)

TABLE 1-3 *(continued)*

FLOORING

Recommendations

➤ Level floor surfaces when possible

➤ Variations in walking surface height highlighted with bright contrasting color (eg, yellow)

➤ Doorsills removed (or reduced with bevel or threshold ramp)

➤ Matte finishes for better traction and reduced glare

➤ Low-pile carpeting for reduced glare and reduced background noise

➤ Light to medium colors for effective light reflectance

➤ No strong color-contrasted borders (may be perceived as a hole to be stepped over for patients with visual/spatial impairments) and simple patterns or no patterns

➤ Rounds by staff to check flooring for fall hazards (eg, easy-to-trip-on turned-up edges on lobby entrance mats) and speedy replacement of identified items

FURNISHINGS

Recommendations

Seating

➤ Varied seating for different user groups

　➤ Loveseats to accommodate obese patients

　➤ Appropriate seating to facilitate transferring

　➤ Armrests that extend to seat edge

　➤ Seat height of 18–19 in

　➤ Seat depth of 18–20 in

　➤ Open space under front of the chair (to allow for patient's placement of feet under center of gravity when rising)

➤ Seating fabrics

　➤ Colors contrasted with floor color

　➤ No bold patterns

Reception Desk/Tables

➤ Wheelchair-accessible reception desk area: 36 in wide (minimum) by 30 in high

➤ Matte finishes to reduce glare

➤ Light to medium colors for increased light reflectance

➤ Rounded corners to avoid bruising

➤ Glass tables avoided

➤ Edges highlighted in contrasting color when appropriate

Examination Tables

➤ Height adjustable to accommodate mobility impaired

➤ Color contrasted to floor

ACCESSIBILITY

Key ADAAG Requirements

➤ No step entrance (eg, level flooring, ramp, or chair lift)

➤ No or low threshold (¼ in without bevel or ½ in with bevel)

➤ Minimum clear opening of 32 in

➤ Lever-style hardware

➤ Maximum 5 lb of force to open or close doors

➤ Appropriate maneuvering space at doors for wheelchair users (measurement varies depending on type of door, floor space, and patient approach)

➤ Accessible hallways (ADAAG requirement varies by spatial configuration and office/ facility type)

➤ 5 × 5-ft turning area for wheelchair turning

➤ Accessible reception desk area (3-ft-wide section at 30 in high)

➤ Grab bars in the bathroom

➤ Accessible sink with opening underneath

TAKE-HOME POINTS

➤ With more people living with disabilities to advanced ages, health care office design should include both building code access requirements and age-friendly design features for enhanced patient access, function, and safety.

➤ Everyone's functional capacity, including staff and patients of all ages, is enhanced when environmental barriers are removed and universal access is introduced.

➤ Practice design should strive to include features that make each office space more universally usable by all patients.

USEFUL RESOURCES

ADA Accessibility Guidelines for Buildings and Facilities (ADAAG) (www.access-board.gov/adaag/html/adaag.htm).

Guenther R, Vittori G. *Sustainable Healthcare Architecture*. Hoboken, NJ: John Wiley & Sons Inc; 2008.

Leibrock C. *Design Details for Health: Making the Most of Interior Design's Healing Potential*. New York, NY: John Wiley & Sons Inc; 2000.

Malkin J. *Medical and Dental Space Planning: A Comprehensive Guide to Design, Equipment, and Clinical Procedures*. 3rd ed. New York, NY: John Wiley & Sons Inc; 2002.

Cornell University, Joan and Sanford I. Weill Medical College. Environmental Geriatrics: Improving Function & Safety [online course] (http://cornelleg.org).

REFERENCE

1. *U.S. Census of Population and Housing, 1997: Census Brief: Disabilities Affect One-Fifth of All Americans*. Washington: Government Printing Office, 1997 (http://www.census.gov/prod/3/97pubs/cenbr975.pdf)

CHAPTER TWO

Lessons Learned: Environmental Redesign in a Geriatrics Practice

Audrey Chun, MD

The Coffey Geriatrics Practice at Mount Sinai Medical Center is dedicated to the care of adults over 65 years old. As a primary care practice, it faces the same constraints of most: infinite need with limited resources, space, and reimbursements. Limited space was identified as a major deterrent to efficient flow and expansion of the practice. We were fortunate to have a generous gift from the Martha Stewart Foundation to support the gut renovation of existing space within the medical center to house our geriatrics practice in the Martha Stewart Center for Living. However, through the process of planning and implementation, several questions came up. How much space is needed? With a limited budget, what should be prioritized? Where does one go for such advice? Our lessons learned highlight the experience of one ambulatory geriatrics practice in an academic institution. We share these tips that we obtained in informal interviews with clinician champions, clinicians, staff, administrators, and nurse care managers before the renovation/move and then 2 years after the experience to reflect on the impact of our office redesign.

OPPORTUNITIES

In addition to the opportunities outlined in Chapter 1, structural redesign specifically improved care for older patients in our practice in the following ways:

1. Improved patient access

   ➤ The new space allows patients direct access from the street to the practice without having to navigate through corridors, stairs, or other practices.

   ➤ Automatic doors allow patients with assistive devices to enter and exit easily.

2. Finishes that consider the needs of older adults

   ➤ Flooring that is slip (and scuff) resistant, even when wet, is essential for a population at increased risk for falls.

   ➤ Surfaces include nonreflective materials, such as stone and wood, to reduce glare.

   ➤ Sound-absorbing wall materials and ceiling tiles decrease ambient noise and allow patients and care providers to communicate with each other more easily.

3. Ergonomically appropriate fixtures, furniture, and equipment

   ➤ Adjustable-height examination tables allow patients of varying heights and physical ability to more easily access the table for a complete evaluation.

   ➤ Sturdy chairs with arm rests extending beyond the face of the leg supports allow patients to stand and sit more easily and safely.

   ➤ Recessed lighting decreases glare and is especially important for those with low vision.

   ➤ Handrails provide support along all corridors.

4. Healing and tranquil environment

   ➤ Although the environment was designed for older adults, the end result is one that would be appropriate for any population. It is an inviting, calm environment that promotes healing. There is little ambient noise, and a smooth flow to the visit decreases the "hospital" feel of the ambulatory visit.

5. Multipurpose rooms

   ➤ Part of the mission of our practice is to encourage patient self-management, healthy living, and education. The redesign included multipurpose rooms for:

      ➤ Group visits

➤ Healthy living activities

➤ Education seminars

➤ Family meetings

➤ Precepting for trainees

6. Optimized flow from registration to checkout

➤ Compared to the previous space, the redesigned space is more efficient, less confusing, and less chaotic. Patients and providers express more satisfaction with the current environment, and it has become an example for other practices within the medical center to consider in their own redesigns.

CHALLENGES

Despite careful planning, certain elements of our environmental redesign resulted in suboptimal interfaces with our patients, staff, and providers. However, adaptation to these challenges has resulted in workable solutions.

1. Storage

➤ Because of budgetary constraints, extra cabinets in the examination rooms were eliminated from the construction. The result was limited space for office supplies needed for patient care (eg, patient forms, gauze, ear loop, suture removal kits, tongue depressors, sheets, patient gowns).

Adaptation:

➤ Additional time is allocated to stock the rooms more frequently than in the previous space.

2. Heavy examination room doors

➤ Examination room doors were designed to meet fire codes and match the interior design of the entire space. However, after the construction was completed we realized that, because of the extra height of the space, the doors were quite difficult to open for many patients.

Adaptation:

➤ Special care is taken to make sure frail elders have assistance with opening the doors when leaving the examination room, or to make sure the examination room door remains open after the visit to allow patients to exit with ease.

3. Rooms of varying sizes

   ➤ One of the highest priorities with the redesign was to increase the number of examination rooms to allow for improved patient flow through the practice and to minimize the need for patients to move from site to site for procedures or additional studies. However, because of space limitations and other space requirements (for load-bearing columns, plumbing considerations, etc), the compromise was to decrease the examination room sizes overall. As a result, some of the rooms are quite cramped if patients arrive with family, caregivers, and assistive devices.

   Adaptation:

   ➤ Accommodating our patients' needs requires the flexibility of our providers to change rooms as needed and the foresight of our medical assistants to consider room size before leading the patient to a room. At times, creative adjustments to the configuration of seating are needed to make sure everyone needed for the visit can be present.

4. Furniture for staff

   ➤ Another consequence of our decision to give priority to the number of rooms over the size of the rooms was the selection of furniture and supplies for the room. Provider desks were small and simple in design to maximize the space available for patients and their assistive devices. However, a telephone, computer, and screen take up the majority of desktop space, with little room for providers to write out prescriptions, sign forms, review records, or place medication bottles for review. Additionally, in some of the smaller rooms, if the examination table is left in the supine position, the door hits the table when opening.

   Adaptation:

   ➤ Computer processing units were mounted to the side of the desks and telephones were wall-mounted to open up the area.

   ➤ Infrequently used supplies and forms were removed and placed in a central storage area for use as needed.

   ➤ Examination tables must be left in a more upright/chair-like position to allow doors to open completely in some rooms.

5. Cramped administrative spaces for staff and providers

   ➤ Since priority was placed on patient examination rooms, the remaining space was divided for administrative use by staff and providers. In some cases, the space was smaller than in the previous design, resulting in some resentment and staff concerns about their ability to do their jobs.

Adaptation:

➤ The redesign provided an opportunity to remove unnecessary items, reevaluate workflow, and reconsider the format of necessary items (eg, could a paper copy be stored electronically and printed only as needed?).

➤ For items or activities that truly could not be accommodated in the originally assigned areas, we identified other common areas.

LESSONS LEARNED

1. Prioritize needs.

   ➤ Given limited budgets, it is unlikely that you will be able to make every renovation desired.

   ➤ Environmental design elements that you are considering for redesign should be ranked according to priority. See Table 2-1 for a list of design considerations.

   ➤ Prioritize based on patient and staff/physician needs and make these clear to all parties.

   ➤ While the experience of this primary care redesign may be beyond the scope of smaller or other types of practices, certain design elements do stand out as higher priorities. Table 2-2 highlights some examples of priorities for practice design by specialty.

2. Communicate effectively.

   ➤ Consider using patient focus groups to understand what patients feel are the biggest obstacles to navigating the practice.

   ➤ Meet with staff and physicians regularly regarding decisions, progress, and changes to the original plans.

   ➤ Address concerns, and be transparent about why some requests may not be accommodated. Better yet, include staff and physicians in important decisions related to the redesign. For example, they may be told, "We have $10,000 and have to choose between new computers for the rooms or adjustable-height exam tables. Which do you think will have the best impact for our practice and patients?"

   ➤ Manage expectations. Provide a realistic vision of changes the practice can expect.

TABLE 2-1 Prioritizing Design Elements in Environmental Redesign

Design Element	Rank
Number of examination rooms	
Size of examination rooms	
Hallways/doors to wide enough to accommodate wheelchairs	
Finishes, eg:	
Matte (nonglare)/nonslip flooring, eg, treated stone and tiles	
Sound-absorbing materials	
Furniture, eg:	
Adjustable-height examination table	
Provider desk	
Patient chairs with armrests, firm cushions	
Chairs with arms that extend beyond face of leg support	
Fixtures, eg:	
Handrails	
Nonglare lighting	
Task lighting where reading is required	
Equipment, eg:	
Hearing amplifiers	
Assistive devices	
Storage, eg:	
Examination room supplies	
General practice supplies	
Administrative space for staff	
Flexible spaces	

3. Map current visit and office flow.

    ➤ Consider whether any of your environmental design changes will affect your current workflow. For example, printers located at the front desk instead of in each room might change how information is communicated to the front desk staff about follow-up appointments and prescriptions.

TABLE 2-2 Example of Design Priorities by Specialty*

EMER = Emergency Medicine
GEN SUR = General Surgery
GYN = Gynecology
URO = Urology
PM&R = Physical Medicine and Rehabilitation
THOR = Thoracic Surgery
ORTH = Orthopedic Surgery
OPH = Opthalmology
ENT = ENT

* Design priorities are from an American Medical Association survey of 415 physicians representing nine medical or surgical specialties where more than 40% of participants indicated that the design element was "necessary."

	EMER	GEN SUR	GYN	URO	PM&R	THOR	ORTH	OPH	ENT
Design Elements									
Seating options with armrests					X		X	X	
Examination room large enough to accommodate assistive devices (eg, caregiver, walker, stretcher)		X	X	X	X	X	X	X	X
Halls wide enough to accommodate assistive devices (eg, caregiver, walker, stretcher, wheelchair)	X		X	X	X		X	X	X
Doors wide enough to accommodate assistive devices	X		X	X	X	X	X	X	X
Office equipment									
Adjustable-height examination tables			X	X	X				
Office materials									
Large-print office forms, patient education materials								X	

(continued)

TABLE 2-2 *(continued)*

	EMER	GEN SUR	GYN	URO	PM&R	THOR	ORTH	OPH	ENT
Office flow practices									
Longer appointment times/specific appointment times for patients with disabilities			X	X	X				
Training for staff related to interactions with older adults and common communication barriers	X			X	X	X			X
Personal appointment reminders			X	X	X	X	X	X	X

4. Be prepared for the systems change that often follows structural change.

   ➤ Although environmental design changes may seem simple or straight-forward, changes can have unexpected consequences to office flow or might even be an opportunity for staff and physicians to consider related design changes that could be implemented at the same time.

5. Mock up the space.

   ➤ Blueprints can be misleading, since people often have misperceptions about what can fit into a given dimension.

   ➤ Before approving any design, it is a good idea to literally outline the area on the floor and place or mark the space for items you want in a room, eg, examination table, desk, chairs, trash bin, soiled utility bin, and examination supplies. Walk in the outlined area and even try pushing a wheelchair in the space to see if you can adequately maneuver in the space.

6. Plan for equipment/furniture that accommodates both patients and staff.

   ➤ With so much attention focused on the patient, it is easy to forget or even dismiss staff and provider needs. However, if physicians and staff are unable to do their jobs efficiently and comfortably, there will be diminished job satisfaction and possibly decreased quality of patient care.

7. Consider materials within the context of how they might affect patients.

   ➤ Costs being equal, consider the impact of your choices on patients. For example, floor tiles of the same price may come in both matte and glossy finishes. The matte finish would be more appropriate for accommodating the vision changes that occur with aging.

8. Don't forget about storage.

   ➤ Both examination room and general practice supplies need to be easily accessible and replenished with reasonable ease. Failure to do so can result in a less efficient workflow.

9. You will not please everyone.

   ➤ Redesign often requires compromises and difficult decisions.

   ➤ Anticipate potential problems and address them early.

   ➤ Communicate your thinking, and be transparent about the reasons for difficult decisions. Most reasonable people will appreciate your efforts.

10. Change is hard, but the final outcome is worth it.

    ➤ Keep the ultimate goal in mind, and know that you are working toward improving care for older adults.

    ➤ Overcoming challenges makes achieving your goals more rewarding.

ACKNOWLEDGMENTS

The Martha Stewart Living Omnimedia Foundation provided generous support through our office redesign and advocating for better care for older adults. Our patients, staff, and physicians have made immense contributions toward continuous improvements in the practice.

CHAPTER THREE

Developing a Plan to Assess Your Practice

Lisa Caruso, MD, MPH

Heidi Auerbach, MD

Ann McDonough, MS, RN

MR ADAMS' EXPERIENCE

Mr Adams is a new patient in Dr Boston's primary care practice. Mr Adams is an 80-year-old man with diabetes and hypertension who was previously getting most of his primary care through specialists. His diabetes and hypertension are poorly controlled and he does not take his medications regularly. He has been falling at home and has had episodes of hypoglycemia. Mr Adams is like many older adults who often have multiple comorbidities such as congestive heart failure, coronary artery disease, and diabetes. These patients with complicated health issues are also at risk for developing geriatric syndromes such as dementia, incontinence, depression, and falls. How should Dr Boston assess her practice and its care of older adults like Mr Adams to best accommodate their needs?

OPPORTUNITIES

Developing a plan to assess one's practice is an important step toward identifying areas for improvement and creating the foundation for improving systems and delivering quality care. Clinical providers, office support staff, patients, and families are all important participants in this process.

Collaborating with patients in a model of patient-centered care can improve patient satisfaction as well as clinical outcomes by addressing what matters most to patients during an encounter.[1] The performance and quality improvement process begins with choosing practice metrics and identifying quality indicators that are important and meaningful to a geriatric population and to the practice staff.

➤ *Improved operations:* Assessment of the practice has the potential to improve efficiency and utilization of personnel and resources.

➤ *Patient satisfaction:* Identifying areas for improvement, especially when taking into account patient satisfaction data, likely will improve patient views of the practice. Knowing how to assess patient satisfaction will make its interpretation clearer.

➤ *Staff satisfaction:* If managed well, practice assessment tools can help improve the practice, staff efficiencies, and satisfaction.

➤ *Improved patient safety and clinical outcomes:* Assessing how providers are following through with evidence-based guidelines can improve the process of care delivery, make adhering to standards easier for the provider, and result in better outcomes for patients.

➤ *Increased reimbursement:* Measurement of quality indicators under Medicare's Physician Quality Reporting Initiative (PQRI) may impact future Medicare reimbursement rates.

➤ *Valuable innovations:* Identifying areas for improvement and making corrections can enhance the workings of the practice and make it a model for other practices to follow.

CHALLENGES

Although there are many advantages to assessing one's practice, obstacles exist but are not insurmountable.

➤ *Time:* Assessments require staff time in the form of meetings to create and implement plans for improvement and data analysis.

➤ *Cost:* Human resources and electronic health records software and database additions may be required to measure quality indicators and their change in a reliable and meaningful way.

➤ *Data management/sustainability:* Assessment of a practice requires ongoing periodic data collection by a designated administrative staff member who can present the data in a format that can be shared with all members of the practice team. This type of resource may not be available, especially in a smaller practice.

➤ *Staff skepticism:* Staff may not see the advantages of the assessment process and may view it as extra work without value.

➤ *Lack of focus:* Vague assessment goals such as "see more patients" or "keep patients out of the hospital" can be tempting to share with staff, but without defined metrics, targets, and processes, goals may remain vague and unobtainable.

➤ *Heterogeneity of health needs in the older patient population:* Careful application of standards is important; for example hemoglobin A_{1c} targets may be different depending on your patient population's age, functional status, and life expectancy.

SOLUTIONS

Many resources are available to guide the assessment process. The Clinical Microsystems workbook, "Assessing, Diagnosing and Treating Your Outpatient Primary Care Practice," provides useful information on strategies to assess and redesign one's practice.[2]

Major principles from this workbook are outlined below. The Useful Resources section at the end of this chapter provides other assessment tool options to consider. Although the process used is not specific to a geriatrics practice, certain measures may be more important when considering how best to care for older patients.

1. Who is involved? It is imperative that the process have a "champion" or a "lead team."[2]

➤ The "champion" is an individual, or sometimes several individuals, in the case of the "lead team," who are committed to the process of assessment and are able to lead the practice toward change and improvement.

➤ The champions are able to get "buy-in" from other members of the practice.

➤ Members of the lead team should reflect the needs of the patients and the practice staff. One of the champions should be a physician who is able to engage his or her colleagues in responding to assessments and implementing clinically appropriate practice changes. Other members should ideally include a nurse and a practice manager.

2. What is the process for identifying potential areas for improvement? The process begins with considering all aspects of the practice and exploring what areas are recognized by either patients or staff as needing improvement. There are many paradigms for framing the process, but overall there are certain key elements.[2]

➤ *Identify* your *patient population and their reported needs.* Understanding the characteristics of your patients, such as average age, common diseases, levels of function, languages spoken, and cultural backgrounds, will help you identify specific needs for subsets of your patient population. For example, if you find that 25% of your patients have limited English proficiency or have significant physical disability or cognitive impairment, then you may want to assess whether your practice is meeting the needs of these patients. Use patient satisfaction surveys, reports from electronic health records, or other databases to gather information and understand your patients' and caregivers' needs.

➤ *Identify staff characteristics and their reported needs.* It is also very important to know the capabilities of the staff, their work hours and areas of interest, and concerns about the practice. Understanding your staff better will help you recognize how best to utilize their skills to improve your practice. Use staff surveys and team meetings to understand your employees' needs and concerns.

➤ *Look at the practice's daily processes.* Throughout this book are chapters addressing many of these areas in more detail. (See chapters 4, 14, and 16.)

  ➤ Paperwork: This would include work flow for handling forms regarding durable medical equipment, medication prior approvals, adult day health programs, assisted living facilities, Family and Medical Leave Act, and guardianship issues. Review the steps involved, who does what, and how to make the process more efficient.

  ➤ Scheduling: Areas to be reviewed include slots available for urgent visits, wait time for new patient and follow-up appointments, and match-up between actual physician time spent with patients and appointment time allotted.

  ➤ Charting: How easily are medications documented, how are scripts called in, and are there readily available forms for conducting geriatrics screening?

  ➤ Telephone call management: What gets triaged and by whom? Are telephone calls answered promptly and courteously? How are after-hours calls handled?

➤ Test results: What is the process for informing patients of laboratory, test, x-ray, and procedure results?

➤ Work flows: Look at the time and steps involved from patient arrival to departure. What goes smoothly and where are the bottlenecks?

➤ *Review practice patterns.* There are elements of the practice related to communication and the overall "culture" of the practice. For example, what are the standards for communicating practice changes to clinicians and office staff?

3. What should be systematically assessed? The data collection on patient characteristics, the conducting of patient and staff satisfaction surveys, and the review of processes should provide a realistic review of what the practice is doing well and what needs improvement.[2] Choose a workable number of measurable indicators to address at a given time. Below are categories of possible metrics to choose from.

➤ Internal systems process measures include metrics such as:

　➤ Wait time for first or third available appointment

　➤ Wait time to see the provider once the patient has arrived at the office

　➤ No-show rate

　➤ Telephone call abandonment rate

➤ Medically related measures can be found in comprehensive lists of quality indicators related to older adults, such as those outlined in the Assessing Care of Vulnerable Elders-3 (ACOVE-3) Project and measures from the Centers for Medicare and Medicaid Services' PQRI.[3] The Useful Resources section at the end of this chapter provides addresses of several useful Web sites. Examples of measures important for older adults include the following:

　➤ Disease-specific standards of care for chronic diseases common in older adults, such as chronic obstructive pulmonary disease, diabetes, and congestive heart failure

　➤ Standards for assessment and management of geriatric syndromes, such as falls, dementia, depression, and urinary incontinence

　➤ Standards for assessment of routine health care maintenance in older adults, such as cognitive and functional assessment, immunizations, and cancer screening

　➤ Standards related to coordination of care, transitions of care, and end-of-life care.

> A practice can identify measures and choose its own standards on the basis of practice priorities. For examples, a geriatrics practice may develop standards for:

> > Discharge communication from inpatient attending physician to outpatient primary care provider within 24 hours

> > Telephone calls to patients within 72 hours after hospital discharge

> > Medication reconciliation at every visit

> > Documentation of advance directives within 6 months of a patient entering the practice

4. How should the changes be implemented?

> Choose two to three measurable indicators that matter in terms of need to improve patient outcomes and clinic processes.

> Gather information regarding these indicators to find out what your current performance is on the indicators you have chosen.

> Develop specific and quantitative target goals. For example, a target goal for medication reconciliation might be 90% compliance at every visit.

> Develop the process for improvement by using your lead team/champion.

> Test the improvement plan and then implement it with a pilot project. Depending on the results, expand it to the entire practice.

> Continue to measure your performance at set intervals and modify processes as needed.

> Share data with your staff regularly to review and celebrate improvements and motivate them for continued process improvement activities.

> Take advantage of performance improvement continuing medical education (CME) as you develop your plans (see the Useful Resources section).

TAKE-HOME POINTS

Evaluating one's practice is imperative in order to know what is working and what needs improvement.

> The process has multiple steps and requires the resources of a lead team and ongoing communication with staff about process improvement measures.

> Just a few indicators at a time should be chosen to make the process workable.

> It is important to recognize that the assessment process is continuous.

> Use the helpful resources that are available (see the Useful Resources section).

USEFUL RESOURCES

Journal articles

Endsley S, Magill MK, Godfrey MM. Creating a lean practice. *Fam Pract Manage.* April 2006 (www.aafp.org/fpm/20060400/34crea.html).

Saliba D, Elliott M, Rubenstein LZ, et al. The vulnerable elders survey: a tool for identifying vulnerable older people in the community. *J Am Geriatr Soc.* 2001;49:1691–1699.

Stock RD, Reece D, Cesario L. Developing a comprehensive interdisciplinary senior healthcare practice. *J Am Geriatr Soc.* 2004;52:2128–2133.

Web sites

American Board of Internal Medicine (ABIM)

➤ Care of the Vulnerable Elderly Practice Improvement Module (PIM): Provides an opportunity for internists to apply some of the core ACOVE measures to their practices while obtaining credit toward maintenance of board certification and receiving (CME) credits (www.abim.org/moc/choose/module/care-of-the-vulnerable-elderly.aspx).

American College of Physicians (ACP)

➤ The Running a Practice section has many tools and references, though some require membership access. There are free links to ACP Internist—Practice Resources, which has catalogued articles on practice management and Quality Improvement News (www.acponline.org/running_practice/).

American Medical Association (AMA)

➤ Physician Consortium for Performance Improvement (PCPI): Lists nine geriatrics performance improvement measures on medication reconciliation, advance care planning, urinary incontinence, and falls (www.ama-assn.org/ama1/pub/upload/mm/370/geriatrics-ws.pdf).

➤ Physician Consortium for Performance Improvement (PCPI): performance improvement measures on transitions of care (www.ama-assn.org/ama1/pub/upload/mm/370/care-transitions-ms.pdf).

➤ AMA Continuing Physician Professional Development (CPPD) Report. In this issue of the newsletter is useful information about performance improvement CME (www.ama-assn.org/ama1/pub/upload/mm/455/cppd22.pdf).

American Society for Quality (ASQ)

➤ The Health Care division offers information on training and conferences to consider, though not specific to the outpatient setting or to geriatrics. The search engine within the Web site allows locating basic information on quality concepts and basic approaches (http://asq.org).

Assessing Care of Vulnerable Elders (ACOVE-3) Project

➤ A set of evidence-based quality indicators covering 26 conditions and 392 quality indicators (www.rand.org/health/projects/acove/acove3/).

Clinical Microsystems

➤ A comprehensive process improvement system for evaluating the performance characteristics of the practice and the steps necessary to develop a plan for sustainable improvements. Refer especially to the Workbook section on Ambulatory Care. (http://dms.dartmouth.edu/cms/) or (www.clinicalmicrosystem.org).

Institute for Healthcare Improvement (IHI)

➤ Under Topics/Office Practices there are helpful sections on primary care access, patient-centered care, and the chronic care model. Under Improvement Methods/Measures there are informative sections defining types of measures and process improvement plans (www.ihi.org).

National Committee for Quality Assurance (NCQA)

➤ Extensive Web site including the Health Care Effectiveness Data and Information Set (HEDIS) performance measures. This link is specific to the Disease Management Accreditation Program and performance measures that are more applicable to the outpatient setting (www.ncqa.org/tabid/98/Default.aspx).

National Quality Forum (NQF)

➤ Includes a list of NQF-endorsed standards with a search option included (www.qualityforum.org/Measures_list.aspx#).

Physician Quality Reporting Initiatives (PQRI)

➤ Link to the Centers for Medicare and Medicaid Services' comprehensive Web site on all PQRI-related information (www.cms.hhs.gov/pqri/).

REFERENCES

1. Wasson JH, Bartels S. CARE vital signs supports patient-centered collaborative care. *J Ambulatory Care Manage.* 2009;32:56–71.

2. Clinical Microsystems. Assessing, diagnosing and treating your outpatient primary care practice. 2001:1–33. http://dms.dartmouth.edu/cms/materials/workbooks/outpatient_primary_care.doc.

3. Wenger NS, Shekelle PG, eds. Measuring medical care provided to vulnerable elders: the Assessing Care of Vulnerable Elders-3 (ACOVE-3) quality indicators. *J Am Geriatr Soc.* 2007;55(suppl 2):S247–S487.

CHAPTER FOUR

Strategies to Improve In-Office and Telephone Communication

John M. Bruza, MD

DR BOSTON'S EXPERIENCE

Dr Boston has been seeing Mr Adams for 2 months now, but is facing challenges in managing his chronic medical conditions. Mr Adams' wife accompanies him to all appointments. Their three children and five grandchildren live out of state, but call often. He is being monitored by a visiting nurse who started seeing him after a fall due to hypoglycemia, which occurred when he took too many of his medications at the same time. Dr Boston works at a small suburban practice affiliated with a community hospital. Her office is staffed by two other physicians, two nurses, and two practice assistants. The office staff is frustrated by having to field multiple phone calls. How do Dr Boston and her team better manage time with patients during office visits? How can time spent during the office visit reduce the number of telephone calls to the practice and improve direct communication with patients and families?

OPPORTUNITIES

Many clinicians caring for older patients struggle with balancing time among seeing patients, completing paperwork, fielding telephone calls for care coordination, returning patients' calls, and fulfilling other clinical and professional commitments. Effective strategies for making the most of one's time in the office must address the broader scope of how the practice functions. Restructuring the outpatient practice with a team-based approach to care coordination can improve triaging of telephone calls to the most appropriate team members and enhance communication with patients and caregivers.

➤ *Improved efficiency:* Reviewing strategies to maximize communication and care when the patient is present during the office visit and creating an effective delineation of roles to better manage telephone calls can reduce repeated callbacks for the same problems.

➤ *Improved care coordination:* Incorporating a team-based approach to the complex task of care coordination can help streamline communication and thereby improve patient care.

➤ *Improved satisfaction:* Patients, caregivers, clinicians, and staff all value a well-managed working relationship.

CHALLENGES

Managing care coordination for medically complex older patients in an efficient and successful manner in the outpatient setting can pose challenges.

➤ The medical complexity of the condition of some older patients and the need to communicate with multiple medical providers across multiple sites of care can be time consuming. Managing complex patients often requires involvement of several care providers and family members.

➤ Patients and caregivers vary in the amount of emotional and practical support they need, which can mean wide variations in the amount of time spent on the telephone or in the office to address their needs.

➤ Inadequate social supports in the home can lead to recurring crises and calls to the office.

➤ Unrecognized caregiver stress or lack of access to resources can place heavy demands on clinicians.

➤ Transportation needs and limits of caregivers' schedules increase the need for telephone management and care coordination.

➤ Reimbursement for telephone medicine and care coordination is currently limited at best, or not feasible in most practices.

SOLUTIONS

Maximize Efficiency During the Office Visit[1]

➤ Have staff prepare charts prior to the visit to ensure that outside tests and reports are available at the time of the visit.

➤ Prepare for the visit by reviewing previous notes, interval telephone calls, and results.

➤ Include appropriate caregivers in the visit (which is very important for patients with cognitive impairment). Consider a teleconference if necessary.

➤ Ensure that medication reconciliation is performed by a medical assistant or nurse at each encounter.

➤ Establish the agenda for the visit by using open-ended questions to be sure that patients and caregivers are given the opportunity to express their concerns.

➤ Manage expectations of what can be accomplished in a single visit and begin setting the agenda for the next visit.

➤ Refer patients to designated health educators available to the practice when appropriate (eg, for disease-specific education such as diabetes, hypertension, continence training techniques, and medication reviews).

Communication

➤ Review how telephone calls are triaged and directed through the office.

  ➤ Triage calls to staff members with the appropriate skill level.

  ➤ Delineate management of calls from community agencies, visiting nursing agencies, hospitals, and physicians.

  ➤ Review telephone scripting and communication skills across staff levels for courteous and responsive behavior. Building trust between patients and staff facilitates effective team-based care.

  ➤ Review telephone call flow at every staff meeting. Review complaints and errors of communication for performance improvement.

  ➤ Consider matching the needs of particularly challenging patients with the skills of particular staff members.

  ➤ Identify the types of calls that would benefit from early involvement of a physician.

➤ Establish how results of tests will be conveyed (letter, call) and by whom (nurse, physician). Avoid the "no news is good news" approach to close the loop on safe and effective communication.

➤ Provide written patient instructions and a current list of medications at each visit (and encourage sharing or providing copies to caregivers).

➤ Respond in writing to questions from caregivers brought to the visit.

➤ Schedule a follow-up visit at a close interval for discussion of major test results and new care plans.

➤ Develop protocols for handling e-mail communication. Many practices have found e-mail to be an effective tool that is convenient, responsive, and welcomed by patients and caregivers. Most clinicians have found that patients are respectful of their time when this mode of communication is adopted.[2]

Access

➤ Consider increasing the frequency of visits according to the complexity of medical and social problems.

➤ Ensure same-day access for urgent visits. Consider setting aside time during each clinic session for "frozen appointments" or flexible time for urgent visits, hospital discharge follow-up, and short-interval visits. Routine follow-up visits and new patient evaluations should not be scheduled in this time slot, and nothing should be scheduled more than 24 to 48 hours in advance. This allows you to accommodate any last-minute needs of your patients. For example, blocking a minimum of 1 hour during a typical 8 hours of your schedule will allow you to accommodate most urgent visits from your patient panel.[3] Alternatively, using a full-time nurse practitioner for urgent visits, hospital discharge follow-up, or short-interval visits can facilitate access.

➤ Consider scheduling telephone hours for patients to call in to speak to their physician. This can be a successful means of managing necessary returned telephone calls and limit telephone tag or repeated calls.[4]

➤ Minimize "bumping" of scheduled appointments out of respect for patients' and caregivers' schedules. For example, institute a policy not to allow cancelation of sessions inside a 6-week window.

Uniformity of Practice

➤ Create a clinical leadership team that regularly reviews practice performance and processes to improve communication in the office. Consider including representative staff from across disciplines.

> Minimize variations in practice among clinicians to improve quality goals, patient safety, and staff morale. The medical director plays a pivotal role in this regard.

> Emphasize an interdisciplinary approach to care in the practice and communicate this to patients and families.

> Educate patients about your practice philosophy and policies through an introductory handout or Web site.

Challenging Patients or Families

> Involve the clinical leadership team in regular discussions and problem solving around challenging patient situations, complaints, or potential problems.

> Refer patients who require above-average telephone care coordination to the clinical leadership team for review and management suggestions.

> Pay close attention to the interactions of patients with all staff members for subtle signs of as-yet-undiagnosed cognitive impairment or mood disorders.

> Recognize when caregivers are stressed and refer them for appropriate support and resources.

TAKE-HOME POINTS

> A team-based approach to managing office visits and between-visit telephone calls is essential for addressing patients' needs and providing optimal communication with patients and caregivers.

> Successful strategies to balance rewarding and necessary physician-patient telephone calls with other clinical and personal time commitments require a process of ongoing assessment and practice improvement.

USEFUL RESOURCES

American Academy of Family Physicians (AAFP)

> AAFP resources for practice transformation (www.aafp.org/online/en/home/practicemgt/transformation.html).

American College of Physicians (ACP)

➤ Running a practice: practice management (www.acponline.org/running_practice/ practice_management/education/).

American Medical Association (AMA)

➤ Caregivers resource guide (www.ama-assn.org/ama/pub/physician-resources/public-health/ promoting-healthy-lifestyles/geriatric-health/caregiver-health.shtml).

➤ Physician resource guide to patient self-management support (www.ama-assn.org/ama1/pub/ upload/mm/433/phys_resource_guide.pdf).

➤ Solutions for managing your practice (www.ama-assn.org/ama/pub/physician-resources/ solutions-managing-your-practice.shtml).

REFERENCES

1. Gullen DJ. Efficiency through effective communication. ACP Core Instructional Series, video presentation. www.acponline.org/running_practice/practice_management/education/ cis.htm.

2. Scherger JE. Online communication with patients: making it work. *Fam Pract Manage.* 2004;11(4):73–74. www.aafp.org/fpm/2004/0400/p73.html.

3. Friedman JP. Physician time management. ACP Core Instructional Series, narrated PowerPoint video presentation. www.acponline.org/running_practice/practice_management/ education/cis.htm.

4. Conomikes G. Improving telephone management in your practice. *Fam Pract Manage.* 2005;12(5):49–52. www.aafp.org/fpm/2005/0500/p49.html.

CHAPTER FIVE

Patient, Staff, and Personal Satisfaction

Heidi Auerbach, MD

Won Lee, MD

Margaret Kelly, BS, RN

MR ADAMS' EXPERIENCE

Mr Adams has been in Dr Boston's practice for 6 months now and received a patient satisfaction survey in the mail. Mr Adams did not complete or return the survey. When Mr Adams comes to the office, he often spends time socializing with the staff, and Mrs Adams depends on the nursing staff to educate her about her husband's medications. The visiting nurse who monitors Mr Adams at home regularly calls the office with updates about his hypertension and diabetes. Mr Adams enjoys coming to appointments because he rarely leaves the house and has little outside contact beyond the staff of Dr Boston's practice. How can Dr Boston assess Mr Adams' satisfaction with the practice? What are the challenges to assessing patient and staff satisfaction? What are some special ways to enhance care for older patients like Mr Adams and improve physician satisfaction?

OPPORTUNITIES

Assessment of patient and staff satisfaction is essential for identifying areas that need improvement in a practice. However, there is debate over the validity and reliability of satisfaction surveys. If designed well and appropriately utilized, satisfaction surveys provide valuable information to guide strategies for improvement and to provide feedback that is beneficial for patients and staff alike.[1,2]

➤ Conducting satisfaction surveys demonstrates to patients and staff that the practice is willing to receive feedback and implement practice improvement measures.

➤ Results of surveys not only show needed areas for improvement, but also highlight what a practice is doing well, which is good for staff morale.

➤ Survey data can be used for a variety of purposes: to fulfill institutional quality improvement and pay-for-performance initiatives, and physician requirements for board recertification.

➤ Improved patient satisfaction can mean increased referrals and volume.

➤ Improvement in staff satisfaction can reduce staff turnover and improve team cohesiveness, which, in turn, will improve practice function and patient satisfaction.

➤ Survey results often reveal problems that might otherwise be ignored or go unrecognized. Feedback from patients can be a powerful tool for staff to appreciate that change is necessary and to focus efforts on quality improvement projects. Seeing and hearing what patients think can be an eye-opener.

CHALLENGES

There are challenges to developing, implementing, and appropriately analyzing patient and staff satisfaction surveys.[1,2]

➤ *Cost/resources:* This includes staff time and supplies. If a survey company is used, costs are higher.

➤ *Time:* Staff must invest time in choosing and developing a survey. In most cases, practices can use previously validated survey instruments. However, implementation and data analyses can be time consuming.

➤ *Limited sample size:* Limited sample size reduces the reliability and validity of the data. Response rates for older patients may be limited if patient characteristics such as health literacy, ability to read surveys due to vision problems, language barriers, cognitive issues, and caregiver stress are not taken into account.

➤ *Wrong questions asked:* Surveys that are not designed properly answer the wrong questions and therefore waste time and money.

➤ *Staff attitudes:* Practices affiliated with large hospital settings often use industry-developed surveys, which may not be tailored to an individual practice and may provide more data than can be analyzed easily. These results can make staff skeptical about surveys or, alternatively (hopefully), motivated to find a better instrument.

➤ *Too much or too little data:* Too much data is overwhelming and hard to process, and too little data makes results difficult to interpret.

SOLUTIONS

If developed, implemented, and analyzed thoughtfully, satisfaction surveys provide important insights about how a practice is functioning. Think of this as a diagnostic tool to determine what parts of the practice are healthy and what parts need treatment.[3] If surveys are well focused, they can provide important information about what patients feel they need from the practice operationally and for best care.

Patient Satisfaction

1. Choose a tool that fits the resources and time available. It may be useful to use different tools at different times or simultaneously depending on the circumstances. Any formal survey needs to be concise and easy to understand and should use a 5- or 6-point Likert scale as well as an opportunity for answers to open-ended questions. See the Useful Resources section for accessing survey examples.[1]

➤ *Telephone surveys:* These may be more time intensive and may not allow for anonymity, but they provide patients with more time to state concerns in greater depth. These surveys may be more appropriate for patients with limited health literacy.

➤ *Focus groups:* It may be hard to get patients to participate, and also there is no anonymity. However, in a group setting, patients may be more willing to speak their minds among fellow patients.

➤ *Listening and observation:* Even one comment may be enough to consider a need for change. Patients often voice complaints more to office staff than to physicians; it is important to know and to keep track of what patients are saying.

➤ *Written surveys:* These surveys can be distributed at the office or by mail. Each has pros and cons. Mailings may be more expensive but have lower yield. Surveys distributed at the office can be time consuming, but are feasible if targeted for a fixed period of time. Patients may not want to complete a survey without anonymity ensured. See patient survey examples on pages 7 and 8 of the Clinical Microsystems Ambulatory Workbook at http://dms.dartmouth.edu/cms/materials/workbooks/oupatient_primary_care.doc.

➤ *Walk in their shoes:* This is an intriguing exercise to see the practice from the patient's point of view. Have staff simulate a visit from start to finish and see the encounter from the patient's vantage point. See the worksheet on page 9 of the Clinical Microsystems Ambulatory Care Workbook at http://dms.dartmouth.edu/cms/materials/workbooks/oupatient_primary_care.doc for more information.

➤ *Online tools:* Older patients are becoming more computer savvy. If they do not have Internet access, it is likely that their children or grandchildren do.

  ➤ Tools such as the patient portal at www.howsyourhealth.org offer patient-reported measures of health issues important to them that go beyond standard survey questions. Results can be used for direct action at the physician visit to improve patient satisfaction. This Web site can also tally results across a practice and help providers understand patient needs on the basis of specific patient characteristics.[4,5]

  ➤ The Web site www.surveymonkey.com permits free online development of questionnaires with collation of results, which can be helpful for larger surveys.

2. Focus on key elements.

It is vital to know what patients think about how the practice is functioning in terms of access and communication, and whether the practice is meeting their needs regarding chronic disease management and physical function.[1,2,6]

➤ *Access:* How easy is it to schedule an appointment, test, or referral? What is the perception of wait time? In a geriatrics practice, it is also important to identify promptness in having prescriptions filled, turnaround time for completing paperwork on such items as durable medical equipment and medication prior approvals, and convenience in getting to the office from the parking lot or public transportation.

➤ *Patient experience:* What do patients think about the medical care they are receiving? Older patients very much appreciate having enough time spent with them to have all of their questions answered. They value a holistic approach with attention to functional and emotional concerns and want health problems addressed and not dismissed as just age-related problems. Questions on quality need to address whether patients' concerns about their health problems and physical function are being addressed by the practice.

➤ *Communication/interpersonal:* Do patients feel that they are treated as individuals, and do they feel that they can easily talk to their providers? Respect, courtesy, understanding, and concern for the patient are common positive attributes patients will remark about on surveys.

➤ *Overall satisfaction score:* It can be useful to follow an overall score over time, but it takes a more in-depth analysis to determine what has caused the score to improve or worsen.

➤ *Open-ended questions:* These allow factors that can affect overall satisfaction to be raised, such as issues with the office space, how bills are handled, and parking concerns.

3. Implement a satisfaction survey

➤ The process of choosing or creating a survey, and then conducting and analyzing results, requires a dedicated team to follow through on every step of the process.

➤ Even if the response rate is low, themes can be identified to act on for practice improvement. Each response should be considered individually to determine what is best for the practice and patients. If a patient has completed a survey with patient-reported measures, even one survey can provide useful information for staff to act on for the individual patient.

➤ Actionable items need to be prioritized, and the team must undergo a process to review and then redesign practice protocols. This may involve review of work flows, time management, services offered, and front-desk communication. See Clinical Microsystems at www.dms.dartmouth.edu for examples of redesign strategies.

Staff Satisfaction

1. Choose a format based on the size of the practice

➤ A written survey may seem too formal in a small practice. Regardless of staff size, it is important to elicit direct feedback. Staff will feel empowered and heard when they are given the opportunity to express their opinions and voice their concerns. This can improve staff satisfaction in and of itself. As with patient surveys, staff survey questions should be designed to answer specific questions that will help target areas for improvement. A staff satisfaction survey example can be found on page 12 of the Clinical Microsystems Ambulatory Care Workbook at http://dms.dartmouth.edu/cms/materials/workbooks/oupatient_primary_care.doc.

2. Surveys should include basic content

➤ Staff morale

➤ Adequate resources to perform one's job well

➤ Stress level

➤ Ease of communication among staff and supervisors

➤ Fairness of staff assessments

➤ Recommendations on whether to suggest the practice to others

3. Obtain informal feedback

➤ Use regular staff meetings to elicit feedback.

➤ Touch base with staff on a regular basis to encourage communication, emphasize openness to share ideas, and admit when there are problems.

➤ Use annual reviews as an opportunity to hear what staff are thinking.

➤ Hold a staff retreat to brainstorm ideas, and review what works and does not seem to be working in your practice. It also functions to enhance office spirit and team building.

Personal Satisfaction: "Practicing Outside the Box"

Although there can be many challenges to providing care to elders and many stressors in helping patients navigate through our complex health care system, taking care of older patients is tremendously rewarding and enriching. Our patients and their families teach us and remind us on a daily basis what being older is all about, and for that we can only respect and admire their courage, fortitude, and resilience. Satisfaction surveys are important and can provide innovative ideas for practice improvement. However, great ideas may also come from spontaneous brainstorming and from creative and generous thinking on the part of staff. Think about what makes your patients special and what gives you and your staff enjoyment and fulfillment in taking care of them. Find time every 6 months or so to reflect on the mission and goals of your practice and to reenergize staff interest and enthusiasm. Below are examples of a few of the ways to enhance your practice by working "outside the box." By doing so, you will likely achieve improved satisfaction from patients and staff and sustain your enjoyment in your practice.

1. Recognize elders as vulnerable individuals. Many elders are isolated and have limited resources and tenuous support systems. Your practice may be their only stable link to the outside world. The goal of activities such as those listed below is to keep patients as independent as possible and to strengthen connections with them and their community.

➤ Establish a patient care fund to be used to purchase items such as water bottles and pill boxes.

➤ Recruit volunteers and solicit donations to help an elder furnish a new apartment.

➤ Create special services such as prefilling pill boxes for patients who are at high risk of medication errors and have no one else to help them.

➤ Solicit donations from staff for gifts to give during the winter holiday season to isolated elders who may have few friends or family.

➤ Encourage staff visits and frequent contact with community agencies, adult day health centers, and assisted living facilities to build relationships and strengthen communication.

➤ Develop a directory of frequently used local community resources for patients and caregivers.

2. Appreciate frailty and illness in this population.   By virtue of caring for an elderly population, practice staff members manage illness and end-of-life issues frequently. Repeatedly dealing with loss can take its toll in many ways and affect patient and staff morale.

➤ Provide support to families and caregivers by sending condolence cards and attending wakes and funerals if possible.

➤ Create a support group for family caregivers.

➤ Set aside time periodically to discuss particularly difficult patient experiences. Allow processing of emotions and purposeful reflection on one's professional mission and goals. Staff and providers often build longstanding and significant relationships with patients and need support as well.

➤ Institute staff appreciation activities. Make time to celebrate and commemorate important life events together. Hold team-building exercises to permit staff to get to know each other on a more personal level. Recognize "heroes" on a monthly basis to highlight staff members who have gone above and beyond for patient care or teamwork.

3. Be creative.   Projects that celebrate aging or patients' talents can highlight the unique and special talents and backgrounds of older patients. Many of these ideas can contribute to the overall décor of the clinic space while allowing patients to feel connected personally to the practice.

➤ Highlight the specialness of your patient population. In urban settings, patients often come from a variety of countries. Hang a map on the wall for patients to mark their country of origin or keep a bulletin board of postcards from patients' travels. Likewise, display patient achievements and important anniversaries or events of historical interest. Include art that portrays elders and different cultures in a positive, inclusive way.

➤ Recognize artistic talents. Display patient-created paintings, photographs, or craft work in the reception area.

4. Involve patients. Involving patients in educational and academic activities can contribute to patients' overall satisfaction and improve care.

➤ *Educational activities:* Display bulletin boards in the waiting room or hold group education classes to highlight common medical topics or related issues such as understanding health insurance. Provide educational videos on common patient or caregiver concerns.

➤ *Research opportunities:* If research studies are available in your practice or in an affiliated institution, enrolling patients or providing information on research studies can contribute to their satisfaction. Many patients appreciate being offered new medical innovations or value taking part in potential medical advances. See the Useful Resources section for ClinicalTrials.gov.

TAKE-HOME POINTS

➤ Evaluating patient satisfaction is an essential part of assessing one's practice. Learn what older patients and their families value and need—work toward improving the practice from their vantage point.

➤ Staff satisfaction is also very important. Understanding staff's perspectives and needs can only help to improve morale and enhance collaboration for practice improvement.

➤ Personal satisfaction also needs nurturing. Take the time to appreciate the specialness of caring for older adults—they can teach us so much. The rewards are immeasurable.

USEFUL RESOURCES

American Academy of Family Physicians (AAFP)

➤ Go to the Family Practice Management link and search for "patient satisfaction." This will lead to several articles, including those referenced below (www.aafp.org).

American College of Physicians (ACP)

➤ Provides sample surveys and also a tip book on patient satisfaction surveys (www.acponline.org/running_practice/quality_improvement/satisfaction_surveys/).

Agency for Health Care Research and Quality (AHRQ)

➤ Helpful resource for patients, with useful information on what patients should be asking providers and what practices should be providing patients to improve patient satisfaction (www.ahrq.gov/questionsaretheanswer/).

➤ A helpful site for accessing survey tools for the ambulatory setting (www.cahps.ahrq.gov/content/products/PROD_AmbCareSurveys.asp?p=102&s=21).

American Medical Association (AMA)

➤ Helpful hints on improving standard metrics of patient satisfaction (www.ama-assn.org/ama1/pub/upload/mm/368/patient_satisfaction.pdf).

Clinical Microsystems

➤ Comprehensive Web site on evaluating/redesigning a practice. Click on Materials, then Workbooks, then Ambulatory Practice, where you will find sample surveys and useful material on processes for practice redesign (http://dms.dartmouth.edu/cms or www.clinicalmicrosystem.org).

ClinicalTrials.gov

➤ A registry of federally and privately supported clinical trials that can be searched by topic and location to provide patients and families with information on clinical trials currently in progress or closed (www.clinicaltrials.gov).

How's Your Health

➤ Comprehensive Web site with patient-centered surveys that can help assess patient satisfaction (www.howsyourhealth.org).

Medical Group Management Association (MGMA)

➤ Listings of potential resources. Most require membership in MGMA, but a few are free PDFs, including a sample survey and helpful hints (http://find.mgma.com/globalcontent.aspx?q=patient%20satisfaction).

SurveyMonkey.com

➤ This is a useful Web site for designing surveys of all kinds (www.surveymonkey.com).

REFERENCES

1. White B. Measuring patient satisfaction: how to do it and why to bother. *Fam Pract Manage*. 1999;6(1):40–44.

2. Thiedke CC. What do we really know about patient satisfaction? *Fam Pract Manage*. 2007;14(1):33–36.

3. Clinical Microsystems. Assessing, diagnosing and treating your outpatient primary care practice. 2001:2. http://dms.dartmouth.edu/cms/materials/workbooks/outpatient_primary_care.doc.

4. Wasson JH, Baker NJ. Balanced measures for patient-centered care. *J Ambulatory Care Manage.* 2009;32(1):44–55.

5. Wasson JH, Bartels S. CARE vital signs supports patient-centered, collaborative care. *J Ambulatory Care Manage.* 2009;32(1):56–71.

6. Epstein RA, Mauksch L, Carroll J, Jaen CR. Have you really addressed your patient's concerns? *Fam Pract Manage.* 2008;15(3):35–40.

CHAPTER SIX

Patient Education Materials

Won Lee, MD

Daniel Oates, MD, MSc

MR ADAMS' EXPERIENCE

Mr Adams is a diabetic and hypertensive patient who does not follow dietary recommendations. His wife has limited English proficiency and does all the food preparation at home. Dr Boston feels there is too little time during visits to talk about dietary changes such as following a low-sodium diet on top of managing Mr Adams' other medical issues. How can patient education materials help Dr Boston address Mr Adams' dietary needs? What are the challenges to using patient education materials? What are some resources for finding patient education materials?

OPPORTUNITIES

Patient education materials can help patients understand common clinical problems. Research suggests that when physicians help patients understand their health problems and their care, patients are more satisfied with that care, physicians are more committed to the health care process, and outcomes of care are improved.[1,2]

➤ *Improved efficiency of practice:* Informative materials for patients to take home or read while waiting can enhance how time is utilized during visits.

➤ *Improved patient satisfaction:* Patients may feel empowered by having information and ways to improve communication with their physician (eg, "Ask Your Doctor" cards).

➤ *Improved staff satisfaction:* Nursing staff, social workers, physician assistants, and dieticians who are available to the practice may be able to use materials to educate patients and caregivers and at times may be more effective than physicians for these educational interventions, as they may be less pressed for time.

➤ *Increased patient compliance:* Clear educational materials can facilitate patients' ability to adhere to recommendations and motivate patients to actively control their health.

➤ *Improved quality of care:* Improving patient adherence through education can improve the perception and actual quality of care. Additionally, patient education can be linked to quality indicators to improve quality of care.

➤ *Standardization of information between providers:* If a patient was given a handout on hypertension by another clinician on a previous visit, this can be used as a frame of reference for future discussions with other clinicians.

➤ *Staff education:* Written materials may also serve to educate providers on topics that they may not be familiar with. For example, not all staff in the practice may be aware of what foods to avoid in hyperkalemia.

CHALLENGES

Despite these benefits, there are practical challenges that may prevent use of patient educational materials.

➤ *Substitution for direct patient communication:* Written materials should not take the place of provider-patient communication, and care should be taken to avoid perception by patients as such.

➤ *Too little time:* The amount of information available can be overwhelming, and reviewing materials can be time consuming.

➤ *Limited space:* Offices may have limited space to display materials for easy use and limited storage space to store extra materials that are not currently being used.

➤ *Cost:* There may be an initial cost to purchase materials or an ongoing expense required to reproduce existing or free materials.

➤ *Diverse patient population:* Some materials may not be available in multiple languages or take cultural differences and varying degrees of health literacy into account.

➤ *Overwhelming to patients:* Patients with multiple medical issues may be easily overwhelmed by being given multiple handouts, which thus may decrease patient satisfaction.

➤ *Applicability:* Materials about certain medical conditions may be difficult to apply to patients with individualized care plans or multiple comorbidities.

APPRAISING WRITTEN MATERIALS FOR PATIENTS

There is a vast amount of educational material available to clinicians, yet these materials vary widely in user friendliness. (See Chapter 30 for additional considerations for health literacy for older adults.) Forty-four percent of US adults read at an eighth grade level or below.[3] Up to 70% of adults 85 years or older have marginal or limited health literacy, and they have limited ability to understand and use health information.[4]

➤ Given these limitations, one needs to ensure that chosen print materials are user friendly for patients.[5]

　➤ Text should be only 50% of the handout/pamphlet.

　➤ Type should be 14 point "plain" font for older adults (it should not be a fancy, designer typeface).

　➤ Text should be in dark print on a light background.

　➤ There should be no text printed over pictures or visual images.

　➤ Materials should use pictures to help emphasize key points.

　➤ Text should not "wrap around" pictures.

　➤ Phrases and bulleted points are preferred over long paragraphs.

➤ Handouts are most effective if one takes time to review them with patients in simple language to give them context for the information provided.

➤ Given these limitations, written materials alone are rarely sufficient to teach new concepts.

➤ Clear communication strategies are effective at improving communication and understanding.[6] Some examples:

  ➤ Avoid the use of jargon in communication.

  ➤ Limit the amount of new information discussed at any one encounter.

  ➤ Stress concrete, specific action steps the patient should take. Consider providing individualized written instructions, which can be done with an electronic health record.

  ➤ Minimize information about anatomy and physiology.

  ➤ Use written materials with pictures to help stress important points.

  ➤ Confirm understanding at the end of encounter by using a phrase such as, "Can you tell me what we have talked about today?"

➤ Get feedback from your patients as to what works well for them and what does not.

SOLUTIONS

➤ Assess existing practice and the specific needs of a clinic's patients, providers, and staff.

  ➤ Identify what patient education resources are already present.

  ➤ Identify gaps in education materials.

  ➤ If an electronic health record is used, determine whether it can be useful as a resource for patient education materials.

➤ Choose which medical conditions are the most applicable to the patient population and what language translations are most commonly needed.

➤ Identify which media will best fit into the practice (ie, handouts, brochures, posters, videos, Web sites, or combination of these).

➤ Determine how much of the budget is allocated to educational materials and estimate the cost of materials needed.

➤ Identify the optimal location to display materials for easy access and space to store extra materials. For example, waiting areas can be utilized for both written and video presentations.

➤ Determine which materials should be used by which staff members, and then organize materials in appropriate locations depending on who will be distributing them.

USEFUL RESOURCES

American Diabetes Association

➤ Most materials in Spanish language. Look under Resources for Professionals (http://professional.diabetes.org/).

American Geriatrics Society

➤ Aging in the Know: includes resources such as What to Ask? Questions for Your Healthcare Provider (www.healthinaging.org/agingintheknow/).

American Heart Association

➤ Web-based information for patients, including recipes, a video library, and information in other languages (www.hearthub.org).

Centers for Disease Control and Prevention

➤ Web-based and printer-friendly materials on healthy aging; includes a section on caregiving resources (www.cdc.gov/aging/index.htm).

Family Caregiver Alliance National Center on Caregiving

➤ Includes resources for caregivers such as fact sheets regarding legal issues and advocacy as well as information in Spanish and Chinese (www.caregiver.org).

National Institutes on Aging

➤ Age Pages: materials on a variety of topics, some in Spanish language (www.nia.nih.gov/HealthInformation/Publications/).

➤ "Talking With Your Older Patient: A Clinician's Handbook": includes useful information and helpful resources for variety of topics such as memory loss, driving privileges, assisted living, and more (www.nia.nih.gov/HealthInformation/Publications/).

National Lung Health Education Program

➤ Information for patients and providers about chronic obstructive lung disease (including inhaler use instructions). Many materials can be formatted in large print; Spanish language and posters are available (www.nlhep.org/resources.html).

National Institutes of Health, National Institute of Neurological Disorders and Stroke

➤ Printable brochures, posters, toolkits, many in Spanish (http://stroke.nih.gov/materials/).

NIH Senior Health

➤ Printer-friendly materials on variety of topics; Web site text can be adjusted for contrast, size, and read aloud (http://nihseniorhealth.gov/).

REFERENCES

1. Schauffler HH, Rodriguez T, Milstein A. Health education and patient satisfaction. *J Fam Pract.* 1996;42(1):62–68.

2. Laine C, Davidoff F, Lewis CE, et al. Important elements of outpatient care: a comparison of patients' and physicians' opinions. *Ann Intern Med.* 1996;125(8):640–645.

3. Kutner M, Greenberg E, Jin Y, Boyle B, Hsu Y, Dunleavy E. *Literacy in Everyday Life: Results from the 2003 National Assessment of Adult Literacy* (NESC 2007-480). Washington, DC: US Dept of Education; 2007.

4. Gazmarian JA, Baker DW, Williams MV. Health literacy among Medicare enrollees in a managed care organization. *JAMA.* 1999;281:545–551.

5. Stableford S. 2008 Health Literacy Institute [conference proceedings]. June 8–11, 2008 Freeport, Maine.

6. Oates DJ, Paasche-Orlow MK. Health literacy: communication strategies to improve patient comprehension of cardiovascular health. *Circulation.* 2009;119:1049–1051.

CHAPTER | **SEVEN**

Mentorship Advice on Building a Geriatrics Practice

John Anderson, MD

DR BOSTON'S EXPERIENCE

Dr Boston has many older adults in her practice and is interested in developing a practice in geriatrics. The local hospital's chair of medicine recognizes that the needs of the community for geriatrics care are significant and growing rapidly, and may exceed the needs perceived by other health system administrators. Dr Boston has not yet met with administrators or community stakeholders to determine how this mandate to develop ambulatory geriatric services will be funded. She enjoys ambulatory practice, teaching, and the prospect of building integrated geriatrics services for her community. Dr Boston wonders what strategies will foster success.

GETTING FINANCIAL AND ADMINISTRATIVE SUPPORT ON BOARD

It is essential to speak directly with the business administrators of your prospective program at the outset. Some considerations may include the following:

➤ Do they share your vision for geriatrics services?

➤ How much of your emphasis will be on primary care?

➤ How much of your emphasis will be on consultation?

➤ Will ambulatory practice space(s) accommodate patients and caregivers plus multiple walkers and wheelchairs?

➤ How accessible to the practice are laboratory and imaging services?

➤ Who will benefit and who may resist establishing this practice?

➤ How much will the organization invest to build or renovate space for this practice?

➤ What is the budget for sustaining this practice over the next 3 to 5 years?

➤ What funding sources are expected to support the practice?

➤ What are the long-range goals for this practice?

You may experience pressure with regard to overhead costs, reimbursement, and incentives for more encounters. These numbers are important, but they may be substantially offset by the revenue that will accrue beyond your practice.[1] Frail older adults require very substantial amounts of medical resources. Downstream hospital and ancillary service revenues plus savings generated through competent care of frail elders far exceed the fees generated by a geriatrician. Is your organization structured in such a way that those who profit from geriatric referrals, diagnostics, and/or hospital admissions can find a way to support your practice? If not, what grants, revenues, and private funding sources are anticipated? Who can you count on to bring in that money? Stakeholders in your practice will include patients, families, physicians who prefer to avoid the complexities of geriatrics care, informal and formal caregivers, and the agencies and service providers to whom you refer patients. Building a geriatrics practice requires suitable space, administrative support, shared vision of those who will collaborate in care, and support from the community that will benefit from the services provided.

NETWORKING

Networking is key to realizing and expanding your vision for the development of a geriatrics practice. Sharing and adapting your goals will enable you to harmonize the interests of your practice with those of the community it serves.

➤ Be visible in your institutions and community.

➤ Eat lunch with your staff and colleagues from other disciplines.

➤ Engage with the community through public speaking, Web site participation, newspaper interviews, and television commentary.

➤ Get to know the "players" who are committed to the growth of geriatrics services. These may include any colleague who will value your primary or consultative care for frail older patients (eg, primary care providers with aging practices) and anyone who has the ear of local hospital, community, or regional governance.

➤ Identify and find common ground with individuals and groups who may resist your interest in establishing a geriatrics practice. They may appreciate your willingness to help with some of their more complex and time-consuming cases.

➤ Offer opportunities for dialogue about collaboration by presenting grand rounds with a panel that may include a medical subspecialist, orthopedist, psychiatrist, neurologist, physiatrist, care manager, and social worker to reinforce your team concept to the community and build relationships for continuing professional collaboration as a geriatrics team.

➤ Reach out on the Web to leaders who have established models for high-quality geriatrics care. A sample of sites is included in the references at the end of this chapter.[2,3]

FIND A MENTOR

As you get to know your staff, someone will offer advice that is timely and useful. He or she may have sympathy for your enterprise and useful perspective on how decisions are made in your organization or within the community. Such a person is a natural mentor. If your personal chemistry and schedules bring you together frequently, you can learn from such a mentor in an informal way. It is also important to identify leaders in your medical community whom you admire and trust. Ask for time to meet and bring an administrative problem list along. Society memberships and conference participation will also provide opportunities to meet mentors. Local and state medical societies, the American Geriatrics Society, the American Medical Association, the Gerontological Society of America, the American College of Physicians, and the American Medical Directors Association have all taken educational leadership in the development of geriatric medicine. You can meet excellent mentors at meetings sponsored by these groups. Travel to look at other geriatrics practices and talk with their directors. Experienced leaders who recognize your sincerity in building a geriatrics practice are often generous with their time and advice.

BUILD AND LEARN FROM YOUR TEAM

Geriatrics practice building is a team enterprise. A large, well-funded practice may support many team members to collaborate at a single site. More commonly, your goal will be to develop close coordination with nurses, nurse practitioners, care managers, therapists, specialists, and subspecialists working from multiple sites for expedited geriatrics diagnostic, therapeutic, and social services. Close working relationships with outpatient therapists, visiting nurses, adult day health providers, social workers, and the local Alzheimer disease association are as important as the ability to expedite referrals to neurology, physiatry, psychiatry, neuropsychology, gastroenterology, ophthalmology, dentistry, audiology, and urogynecology. You can build teamwork and create educational opportunities by meeting at regular intervals and providing time for interdisciplinary case review. As your organization grows, you will participate in hiring new staff. Bringing in talented and enthusiastic people will do more to define the quality of your enterprise than any other activity. Ask each prospect to describe his or her dream job and discuss how much of this vision might be realized through participating in the geriatrics practice your group is building. Every member of your team brings unique perspective and talents. As the team matures, consider bringing on a geriatrics care manager to optimize the coordination of medical and social services vital to good geriatrics practice.

CHANGE HATS AND BE A MENTOR

Mentorship and experience make us better. There is stimulation and satisfaction to be found in broadening our work experience and teaching skills to others. Lateral professional moves within systems add perspective on different practice and organizational styles. Participation in PACE (Program for All-Inclusive Care of the Elderly) programs, acute geriatrics inpatient care, palliative care, and nursing home medical directorships will each inform and enrich your capacity as a leader in geriatrics. Enjoy the challenge of sharing your skills through dialogue and collaboration with less experienced health care providers. This aspect of mentorship will also diversify the opportunities you can offer new and prospective colleagues who may want the practice of geriatrics to be only part of their job description.

THE ROLE OF QUALITY

Concentrate on the quality of your geriatrics services and you will soon have more eager patients (and caregivers) than you can make time for. These satisfied patients will build (and fund) your growing practice. Institutional, like political, progress is incremental—often practically glacial. As a geriatrician, the services you help build for your organization and community will be increasingly valued. Geriatrics ambulatory care will be pivotal in developing efficient, effective support systems for transitions to and from hospitals, homes, and extended-care facilities. While "perfect" may be an enemy of "good," quality matters most.

PASSION AND PERSISTENCE

Be flexible. Do not be afraid to compromise, improvise, and adapt as your team grows. In their seminal research on qualities of successful companies, Peters and Waterman wrote, "The top performers create a broad, uplifting, shared culture, a coherent framework within which charged-up people search for appropriate adaptations."[4]

Hold fast to your vision, but let it evolve in the face of both obstacles and opportunities. And learn to repeat yourself. There is always competition for resources among medical, surgical, and other services. By being patient and positive and staying "on message" to make certain that organization leaders and practice colleagues understand your goals, you will maximize the prospect of (re)presenting your plan and (re)stating your needs at a time when those who have the power to help you effect them will understand that your vision is in harmony with their own.

TAKE-HOME POINTS

➤ To build ambulatory geriatrics, be explicit at the outset with your leadership and financial administrators about goals, space, location, staffing, and funding.

➤ Build and learn from your multidisciplinary team through collaboration, regular team meetings, grand rounds presentations, case review, and careful hiring.

➤ Natural mentors may be found in your hospital cafeteria, but be sure to look outside your organization for the expertise of leaders in your medical community and to the models and advice of recognized geriatrics authorities at medical meetings or on the Web.

➤ Be prepared to repeat yourself so that your goals can be heard when others with resources to help are prepared to act.

➤ Remain flexible. Improvise, compromise, and adapt to the needs of your community and to whatever obstacles may arise as you pursue your organization's vision for a high-quality multidisciplinary geriatrics practice.

USEFUL RESOURCES

American College of Physicians (ACP)

➤ Search for "geriatric ambulatory care" (www.acponline.org).

American Geriatrics Society

➤ (http://www.americangeriatrics.org/health_care_professionals/education/
education_programs_products/).

American Medical Association

➤ Search for "geriatrics" (www.ama-assn.org).

American Medical Directors Association

➤ Search for "events" (www.amda.com).

REFERENCES

1. Dang S, Baker G, Lipschitz DA. Financial effect of a hospital outpatient senior clinic on an academic medical center. *JAGS.* 2002;50:1621–1628.

2. UCLA Geronet: Health & Aging Resources for Higher Education. www.geronet.ucla.edu/centers/acove/.

3. University of North Carolina at Chapel Hill, Division of Geriatric Medicine, Center for Aging and Health. www.med.unc.edu/aging.

4. Peters TJ, Waterman RH. *In Search of Excellence: Lessons from America's Best-Run Companies.* New York, NY. Harper and Row; 1982.

CHAPTER EIGHT

Opportunities for Professional Development

Ilona Kopits, MD, MPH

DR BOSTON'S EXPERIENCE

Dr Boston works in a suburban practice affiliated with a community hospital. Her office is staffed by two other physicians, two nurses, and two practice assistants. Dr Boston has 1 week available for continuing medical education (CME) opportunities but is unsure how to best utilize that 1 week per year. She is also looking to develop other professional and educational skills in areas such as practice management and quality improvement. What opportunities exist for professional and educational development?

While there are many CME opportunities for primary care physicians, nurses, and other staff, few focus solely on geriatrics outpatient practice management and improvement. This chapter will outline some opportunities and information for further education and improvement of current practice models.

OPPORTUNITIES

As the population continues to age, the development and improvement of geriatric outpatient practices will be imperative for the future of health care. Primary care physicians need guidance not only in medical care of the elderly, but also in the delivery of care.[1] Creating and maintaining these practices to adapt to current medical practice, costs, and access issues requires constant reevaluation and learning. This is easier said than done. Community-based internists, geriatricians, and family physicians are those most in need of CME in geriatrics management. However, they also face the greatest barriers, in terms of time and money, to access these opportunities. CME programs that use "active-mode learning," a method that involves interactive, targeted techniques such as small group sessions, toolkits, and feedback to physicians, are often most effective in changing practice. This type of CME, however, is often more expensive and more difficult to access, leading some physicians in the community to remain uninterested in the topic.[1]

Conferences

- American Academy of Ambulatory Care Nursing: Annual Conference: www.aaacn.org (under "events").

  - Past sessions on "Train the Trainer" have focused on geriatrics.

    - Competency in geriatrics will be included in next competency document.

- American Academy of Family Physicians (AAFP): Annual Scientific Assembly: www.aafp.org/assembly

  - More than 200 CME courses are offered on a variety of topics, including updates in practice management.

- American Geriatrics Society (AGS): Annual Scientific Meeting: www.americangeriatrics.org

  - Described as the premier educational event in geriatrics, the meeting provides the latest information on clinical care, research on aging, and innovative models of care delivery.

  - Some AGS state affiliates post information regarding local educational meetings through this Web site.

- Institute for Healthcare Improvement: Annual International Summit on Redesigning the Clinical Office Practice: www.ihi.org/IHI/Programs/ConferencesAndSeminars/11thAnnualOfficePracticeSummitMarch2010.htm.

  - Topics include office design, staffing, group visits, access, specialty care, chronic care models, the medical home, and more.

Online CME

- American Academy of Family Physicians: CME Center: https://nf.aafp.org/CME/CmeCenter.

  - Practice Enhancement Forum (online course)

➤ Measuring Evaluating Translating Research Into Care (METRIC)
Module: Geriatrics—Improving Patient Care

➤ Assess practice performance through chart audits that sample key
indicators of high-quality care for geriatric patients.

➤ Evaluate the structure and processes of one's practice.

➤ Select and implement at least one practice improvement intervention to improve care of geriatric patients.

➤ Perform a second assessment of practice performance after
implementing the practice improvement intervention(s).

➤ Summarize the effects of practice improvement on your care
of geriatric patients and patients' outcomes to help you decide
whether this improvement will be a permanent part of the
practice.

➤ American Board of Internal Medicine (ABIM) Practice Improvement
Modules: www.abim.org/moc/.

➤ Modules are Web-based tools to develop quality improvement in practice
with geriatric topics such as Care of the Vulnerable Elderly. Completion
can be applied to maintenance of internal medicine certification.

➤ American College of Physician Executives: www.acpe.org.

➤ Offers useful conferences and online courses on leadership development and management skills.

➤ American Geriatrics Society: ongoing programs in various geriatric topics:
http://www.americangeriatrics.org/health_care_professionals/education/
certification_and_training/ and http://www.americangeriatrics.org/health_
care_professionals/education/courses_conferences_grants_awards/

➤ Includes a link to Geriatrics Review Syllabus (GRS), which is a comprehensive review of geriatric medicine and offers a way to earn lifelong
learning points for those enrolled in the American Board of Internal
Medicine Maintenance of Certification program.

➤ American Medical Association: www.ama-assn.org/ama/pub/
physician-resources.shtml.

➤ CME information includes an archive of webinars addressing topics
such as performance improvement CME.

➤ Institute for Healthcare Improvement, Open School and professional
development: www.ihi.org/IHI/Programs.

➤ Open School

➤ Online courses are offered to students in all health
care professions.

➤ Current courses include patient safety, quality improvement, and operations management.

➤ Professional development

➤ Several programs are focused on safety, quality, and leadership.

USEFUL RESOURCES

AAFP Resources for Practice Management

➤ (www.aafp.org/online/en/home/practicemgt/transformation.html).

➤ Quality improvement resources.

➤ Performance measurement and pay for performance.

American College of Physicians

➤ A section of the Web site is devoted to running a practice and includes such topics as practice management, quality improvement (with a section on geriatrics), and the patient-centered home. Includes resources and CME activities (www.acponline.org/running_practice/).

Clinical Microsystems

➤ Provides strategies for clinical care redesign. Includes modules to review and also offers a program on "coach the coach" training involving online and in-person training (www.dms.dartmouth.edu/cms/events/).

National Association of Geriatric Education Centers (GECs)

➤ Provides contact information for all of the current GECs in the country. Most state/regional GECs have Web sites with information on educational opportunities and materials and a calendar of events on geriatric-focused topics for health care professionals (www.nagec.org).

Portal of Geriatric Online Education (POGOe)

➤ Geriatric Practice Improvement, or "Things I Wish Someone Would Have Told Me When I Started" (www.pogoe.org/product/18966).

➤ Modules regarding improvements in office efficiency and cost-effectiveness, geriatric billing and coding, and innovations in practice.

➤ Overall objective: to help learners "gain novel and necessary information to establish an efficient and effective geriatric practice or to improve their present geriatric practice."

REFERENCE

1. Thomas DC, Johnston B, Dunn K, et al. Continuing medical education, continuing professional development, and knowledge translation: improving care of older patients by practicing physicians. *J Am Geriatr Soc.* 2006;54:1610–1618.

CHAPTER NINE

Getting Your Staff on Board

Elizabeth Eckstrom, MD, MPH

YOUR PATIENTS' EXPERIENCE

You have had a successful primary care practice for almost 15 years and have enjoyed the vast rewards of loyal and grateful patients who have thrived under your care. However, your patients are growing older, and you are finding it increasingly difficult to keep the practice flowing smoothly while attending to their needs. This week, Mrs Johnson complained of her usual headaches and knee arthritis but took an extra 10 minutes to get to a room because she was moving more slowly than usual. Mr Ross lost his charming composure when he admitted that he just couldn't continue to care for his cognitively impaired wife. You found yourself becoming tense and impatient until you realized you had been yelling at Mr Scott because he couldn't hear you otherwise. Mrs Cartwright's blood pressure has suddenly become very high—and it took you an extra 20 minutes to discover that it was because she has been forgetting to take her pills. You wonder what you can do to better utilize your environment, practice team, and electronic resources to care for your older patients.

OPPORTUNITIES

As the American population ages, so do the practices of many primary care clinicians. We may recognize that our clinic staff must have special competencies related to geriatrics, but there are many challenges to enhancing the geriatric flavor of a busy primary care clinic. This chapter will discuss practical ways to enhance teamwork and work flow around the care of older adults, and offer suggestions for improving efficiency of scheduling and clinic access.

First and foremost, all staff members who assist in caring for older patients must believe their work is valued, rewarding, and feasible. As we worked to redesign our own clinic to be more geriatric-friendly, we looked for staff members who already had a geriatrics interest to innovate and help bring other staff on board. One nurse care manager in the practice had a strong interest in older patients and voluntarily participated in continuing education hours on dementia, insomnia, and other geriatrics topics. In addition, I had the opportunity to assist in hiring a new medical assistant for the practice who would be a champion for geriatric patients. I wondered how to maintain sensitivity to the needs of the bigger practice, while steering interview questions in a way that could elicit passion about the particular rewards and challenges of working with older patients. This did not turn out to be difficult; Jody, one of our early applicants, was a recent graduate who professed a strong interest in geriatrics. When I asked her how this developed, she told me that her grandmother had developed dementia and came to live with her family when she was a teenager. Jody would paint her grandmother's fingernails while her grandmother told her stories of her own youth—capturing the heart of this teenager while participating in a normal teen activity. This translated quickly into very patient-centered, compassionate care of our patients, and Jody is now a staunch advocate of superb elder care.

However, we were not done with our geriatric redesign. Our clinic pharmacist teaches pharmacy students and residents and was willing to add geriatrics content to the curriculum, so pharmacists became a vital part of our team, teaching our residents the complexities of geriatric pharmacology and doing medication reviews with our older patients. A retired clinical psychologist who joined our monthly teaching sessions gives us practical tips on the mental health issues our patients face. By seizing opportunities and finding the right team members, we have fostered a strong interprofessional commitment to providing excellent geriatric care throughout the practice.

Geriatrics has unique challenges to clinic efficiency that require flexibility on the part of team members. Listed below are several of the more common challenges, together with some practical solutions that most practices could implement today. The remainder of the Staffing and Human Resources section of this book provides more details and examples of how to ensure a practice can meet the needs of its older patients while maintaining excellent staff engagement and efficiency.

CHALLENGES AND SOLUTIONS

1. Geriatric patients take more time. There is no way to get around this.

Solutions:

➤ Room geriatric patients closest to the waiting room so they can walk the shortest distance. It is much easier for clinic team members to walk further to accommodate the patients.

➤ Place an electric table in one examination room close to the waiting area. It will be easier for the medical assistant to get the patient onto the table.

➤ Have medical assistants carry the "pocket talker" (handheld amplification device) in their pockets and pull it out as soon as hearing difficulties become apparent, rather than shouting or repeating things. Patients' faces light up when they realize they can hear someone clearly, possibly for the first time in years.

2. Geriatric patients have more complex medication lists.

Solutions:

➤ Give patients a printout of the current medication list while they are in the waiting room, and ask them to correct it on the paper while they wait. When the medical assistant completes medication reconciliation in the room, the updated list will help speed the review.

➤ Keep a list of medications to be avoided or used with caution with older adults in a prominent place in the work area. It will help remind everyone on the team to reduce the use of risky drugs.

3. The goals of care for geriatric patients are not always to get better. Often they are more akin to preserving function, so staff may find it hard to maintain a cheerful presence when seeing so much frailty.

Solutions:

➤ During twice-monthly team meetings, we dedicate some time to sharing success stories of our patients. This week an older woman, depressed after her husband's death, had gotten back to her crafts and brought a stuffed animal for a staff member's new baby.

➤ Have all team members participate in setting realistic goals. For example, if a medical assistant notices that an older woman cannot stand from the chair without using her arms, the assistant can discuss exercises to improve this.

4. Some days are really bad days.

Solutions:

➤ At each team meeting, everyone on the team—faculty, residents, care management, front office staff—can share their personal efficiency tips. This often teaches us all new tricks and helps us standardize what is working well across the team.

➤ If a beloved patient has died, giving staff a few minutes to share a story about the patient and sign the sympathy card can be very therapeutic.

5. Providing good geriatric care requires constant attention to complexity.

Solutions:

➤ Our team engages in at least one continuous quality loop at all times (plan, do, study, act). These range from a concerted effort to improve our rate of completion and documentation of advance directives, to improving the efficiency of handling patient messages received via our electronic record. The entire team develops these together and determines how to measure success.

➤ Provide team members with protocols to increase efficiency. If the patient lists incontinence or urinary symptoms as a new complaint, a urine dip could be automatic. If the patient has a history of urinary retention or is a man with a diagnosis of benign prostatic hypertrophy, a bladder scan could be part of the standard protocol. If the patient is having problems hearing, the medical assistant could automatically check for ear wax. If the patient complains of dizziness, orthostatics and an ear check could be part of a standard protocol. Once medical assistants learn the protocols, they feel empowered by their level of input.

➤ All team members should become facile in performing basic geriatric screening tests such as the Get Up and Go, Mini-Cog, and geriatric depression scale.

➤ Some forms should be readily available in the examination rooms, including handicapped driving permit forms, home health referrals, and advance directives.

Getting your staff on board is the first and most important step in designing an elder-friendly practice. It requires attention to the details of the clinic environment; focused, specific training in geriatric principles; and attention to having the right resources at your fingertips. In addition, one must always focus on the patients to energize team goals to provide optimal geriatric care. For example, Grace, who lost her husband to Lewy body dementia earlier this year, glows with affection when Jody checks her in and spends a couple extra minutes asking whether she has started volunteering (she has, with a local theater group). Clarice rates her pain as 10 of 10 when asked, but she grasps the residents' hands in a grateful thank-you for listening to her stories. Nora shares a CD of a record she made during World War II to support the US troops, and the whole team appreciates this lovely voice of a bygone era. Sharing these types of events helps remind the entire team of the great rewards we receive in caring for our geriatric patients.

CHAPTER TEN

Staff Development

David B. Reuben, MD

Brandon Koretz, MD

To accommodate the needs of older persons and provide high-quality care, a practice requires an organized data system (eg, an electronic health record), a workflow that is efficient yet comprehensive, and a team-based approach to patient care. This chapter will focus on principles of staff development and will provide examples of specific tasks that staff can carry out depending on their skills and training. Training, however, is of value only if there is a context in which skills and knowledge can be implemented to improve patient care. In other words, the benefit of tasks that staff perform must be visible to both staff and clinicians and be viewed as worth sustaining. In addition, the value of a prepared, proactive staff is dependent on having monitoring and corrective mechanisms in place to ensure the consistent and accurate completion of tasks. This entire process begins with a set of principles for how to relate to staff and to redefine their roles. It has been noted that improving the quality of relationship among practice staff members can improve health care quality.[1]

CREATING A COMMON FRAMEWORK

The first step in developing staff is to create a culture of teamwork (see Chapter 11: Team Building and Team Dynamics). Staff must view their work as not simply showing up for a job. Rather, they need to feel that they are an integral component of a mission to provide high-quality care for older persons. This concept must be communicated to staff, and every action of each professional and staff member must reinforce it. Ways to accomplish this include the following:

➤ At employment interviews for new staff, emphasize the team approach and discuss how the prospective employee will collaborate with other team members.

➤ Dedicate time to team-building experiences; mark special occasions to permit team members to get to know each other more personally.

Implicit in establishing this culture is the need for communication that is bidirectional between health professionals and staff. Policies and procedures need to be shared among staff and professionals at regular, frequent meetings (at least monthly). The agendas for these meetings should reflect input from both the professionals and the staff. Moreover, the voices of the staff need to be heard at the meetings. Frequently, nonphysician staff members are in relatively powerless positions and may be reluctant to participate actively, much less disagree with physicians. It is the meeting leader's responsibility to ensure the engagement of all staff members. In some practices, a team member other than the physician (eg, a nurse or office manager) may lead the meeting or the facilitator may rotate among team members. Patient evaluations of the practice should be shared with team members and strategies to address concerns developed with team input.

These cultural and communication strategies are important steps to empowering staff and having them take ownership of their responsibilities. Staff must continually seek to improve the work they do and to become more effective in fulfilling their roles and facilitating the care provided by the team. Such empowerment has been a hallmark of the airline industry, where any employee has the ability to stop a flight when a danger is suspected.

When such an environment is present, training of staff can be most effective. Staff development requires that staff learn the "what, how, and why" of their work. If they know the "why," staff can often contribute to the "how" by providing valuable suggestions about where to incorporate these tasks into their workflow. Moreover, understanding why these tasks are being performed will facilitate "buy-in" and help staff become more alert about what an abnormal or borderline test might mean. Tasks that are important in the care of older persons (eg, ear lavage or measuring postural blood pressures with the patient lying and standing) require specific training that can be led by a nurse practitioner or a lead nurse. Once staff are trained, their performance must be monitored by periodic performance appraisals to ensure accuracy, consistency, and value in the patient care process. If errors are detected, then remediation is needed. This begins with feedback that is timely, specific, and directed toward the behavior rather than the person. For example, rather than saying, "You're not doing a good job recording the medication list," a better approach would be, "On Mrs R, the medications were recorded correctly but the frequency of administration was not recorded." Similarly, the value of staff-performed tasks should be periodically reviewed. If a task is not contributing to better quality of care (eg, a physician always rechecks postural blood pressure readings), it should be discontinued.

For several reasons, staff development is a continual process. Over time, staff performance often slips, requiring refresher training. In addition, new approaches and tasks emerge that require additional training. Finally, staff members leave and replacements must be trained.

ADDRESSING UNIQUE ISSUES OF OLDER PATIENTS

With proper training, staff can take larger roles in assessment and monitoring of older persons with specific conditions or problems. Staff can administer self-report questionnaires, ask specific questions about conditions, and perform standard tests. Self-administered, previsit questionnaires (see Chapter 13: Geriatric-Friendly Forms) can briefly screen for almost all geriatric conditions (a notable exception is dementia). However, staff may need to distribute these at the time of the visit check-in so that patients and their proxies can complete them in the waiting room.

In addition, staff can ask specific questions and perform standard tests to identify and monitor the conditions listed in Table 10-1. Staff can also facilitate assessments by clinicians by performing tasks such as:

➤ Assisting patients to undress and dress and get on the examining table

➤ Removing dressings so that a wound can be inspected (and redressing it)

➤ Performing ear lavage to permit viewing of the tympanic membrane

TABLE 10-1 Conditions for Which Staff Can Take Standard Actions

Condition	Test or Task That Staff Can Administer
Visual impairment	Snellen eye chart
Hearing loss	Whisper test or audioscope
Malnutrition	Weight and height (body mass index)
Polypharmacy	Medication review and update of medication list
Chronic illness	Update problem list
Fall risk/immobility	Timed Get Up and Go test, postural blood pressure
Urinary incontinence	Postvoid residual, urine dipstick
Cognitive impairment	Mini-cog or mental status screening
Depression	PHQ-9
Diabetic neuropathy	Monofilament testing, blood glucose check/point of care HbA_{1c}

TABLE 10-2 Conditions for Which Staff Can Provide Specific Education

Condition	Training That Staff Can Provide
Urinary incontinence	Kegel exercises, bladder retraining
Falls	Balance exercises
Nocturnal leg cramps	Stretching exercises
Congestive heart failure	Daily weight monitoring

Finally, staff can be trained to provide patient education materials and review them with patients and families. In addition, staff can provide specific education for conditions such as those shown in Table 10-2.

USEFUL RESOURCES

UCLA Geronet: Health & Aging Resources for Higher Education. For healthcare professionals: office forms (www.geronet.ucla.edu/centers/acove/office_forms.htm).

Reuben DB, Roth C, Kamberg C, Wenger NS. Restructuring primary care practices to manage geriatric syndromes: the ACOVE-2 intervention. *JAGS*. 2003;51:1787–1793.

Ganz DA, Fung CH, Sinsky CA, et al. Key elements of high-quality primary care for vulnerable elders. *J Gen Intern Med*. 2008;23(12):2018–2023.

Snellen Eye Chart (www.amazingeye.com/files/snelleneyechart.jpg).

Timed Get Up and Go Test (www.hospitalmedicine.org/geriresource/toolbox/pdfs/get_up_and_go_test.pdf).

Instructions for the Mini-Cog test (http://geriatrics.uthscsa.edu/tools/MINICog.pdf).

Saint Louis University Mental Status Examination (http://medschool.slu.edu/agingsuccessfully/pdfsurveys/slumsexam_05.pdf).

Personal Health Questionnaire Depression Scale (PHQ-9) (http://patienteducation.stanford.edu/research/phq.pdf).

REFERENCE

1. Lanham HJ, McDaniel RR, Crabtree BF, et al. How improving practice relationships among clinicians and nonclinicians can improve quality in primary care. *Joint Commission J Qual Patient Saf*. 2009;35(9):457–466.

CHAPTER ELEVEN

Team Building and Team Dynamics

Mahnaz Ahmad, MD, MS

"A team is a group with a specific task or tasks, the accomplishment of which requires the interdependent and collaborative efforts of its members.[1]"

If a clinic practice is established, it likely has a culture and roles already well defined. Generally, in any clinic venue, everyone knows who will best organize the holiday party and who is best at keeping track of supply needs. But as you work to "geriatricize" your practice, you will undoubtedly find that some of the teamwork needs are not being met. It is worthwhile to explicitly craft your team to meet the care needs of your older patients, and in doing this, understanding the principles of team building will help you.

Some disciplines embody team building and team dynamics more than others, and geriatrics has appropriately embraced the team concept. An interprofessional team brings together medicine, nursing, social work, and other professions to provide high-quality, evidence-based patient care. As a clinic team grows to include many health professions, new ideas can be shared or generated from the input of diverse team members.[2]

Experts define a successful team as having 10 characteristics[3]:

1. Clear goals that everyone understands, including why the team was formed and how the team functions

2. Defined roles that clearly work together to accomplish the outcome

3. Open and clear communication

4. Effective decision making that is acceptable and meaningful

5. Balanced participation that creates a division of labor according to the skills of individual team members

6. Valued diversity where differences are acknowledged and appreciated as resources and not viewed as hindrances. This transcends typical differences such as race, gender, and ethnicity.

7. Conflict resolution without fear or intimidation

8. Positive atmosphere that allows team members to trust and collaborate with each other even when there are differences of opinion

9. Cooperative relationships that allow team members to appreciate each other for what they bring to the project

10. Participative leadership where the leader is more of a coach or mentor playing an equal role in responsibilities (not a top-down authoritative leader). The leadership may vary depending on the specific task at hand. Many physicians have grown accustomed to being a dominant leader and may need to hone listening and reflective skills to become a more participative leader and team member.

Teams are both dynamic and versatile. The coming together of different disciplines is an asset but can also be challenging. As a clinic team is formed, you may expect it to go through the normal "life cycle" of a team[4]:

➤ *Forming:* a diverse group of people with a common commitment

➤ *Storming:* expression of views with variable consensus and dissent

➤ *Norming:* cooperation between team members

➤ *Performing:* based on a foundation of familiarity and trust building

➤ *Mourning:* accomplishment of team objectives and disbanding (this will not happen for clinic teams that continue to work together).

OPPORTUNITIES

When a team is effective:

➤ Enriched experiences and solutions to problems result because a diverse group of individuals with different backgrounds and expertise are focused on solving a unique clinical situation.

➤ Barriers, pitfalls, and concerns can be identified early.

➤ Solutions and results are often unique and unexpected—and better than you could have thought of yourself.

➤ The clinic operates more efficiently.

➤ Work is not duplicated.

➤ The entire team can take credit for clinic successes.

➤ There are better outcomes and higher satisfaction of team members and patients.

CHALLENGES

Challenges to proper team development include the following:

➤ Some team members may initially be attention grabbers, evaders, or blockers.

➤ Sometimes it is difficult to get institutional and/or administrative buy-in for team training and growth.

➤ Team members may need to enhance skills in active listening.

➤ Team members may have different priorities and may fail to see the common vision.

➤ There is not always an effective leader.

➤ Team development takes an investment in financial and human resources as well as time.

SOLUTIONS

Some solutions for overcoming challenges and developing effective teams include the following[5]:

➤ Hold team-building activities to let team members get to know each other personally. Spend time getting acquainted by sharing favorite hobbies, quotes, or other personal touches. Often a retreat outside the clinical setting can work wonders to establish and enhance team rapport.

➤ Agree to focus on the team goals, eliminating extraneous chatting and all but the most urgent outside requests during team meetings.

➤ Practice clear and respectful communication among all members of the team. At first this may mean specifically asking for opinions of quieter team members, and stopping more vocal team members from interrupting. As the team matures, all members will feel more confident offering suggestions. This is termed an *autonomy-supportive environment*. If a team is having difficulty making the leap to this environment, videotaping and reviewing a couple of team meetings can often expose the changes that need to happen.

➤ Set goals—both individual and group, short term and long term. This could be anything from decreasing wait times for patients to improving percentages of patients who reach diabetic targets.

➤ Set priorities—think of quality, satisfaction, and economic successes. Always keep the ultimate goal of improved patient care and outcomes in focus.

➤ Choose roles for team members with careful consideration of their skill set and how they will interface with the team agenda. Avoid creating a "group of individuals" and focus on making a "team." One study pointed out that the optimal size of a team is six members, and more than 12 would be considered too large. If your clinic is large, you may want to form multiple teams.[6]

➤ Agree on accountability for outcomes, and reward good efforts.

➤ Check in frequently with your team, not only when there is a concern but also as a part of process evaluation.

➤ Be respectful of time—keep each team meeting to its designated schedule.

Good teamwork is essential to providing optimal care to older patients. Though it requires up-front commitment and energy to establish a well-functioning team, the results are worth the effort—individually and for the entire practice.

USEFUL RESOURCES

Wise H, Beckhard R, Rubin I, et al. *Making Health Teams Work.* Cambridge, MA: Ballinger Publishing Co; 1974.

John A. Hartford Foundation Inc. GITT: Geriatric Interdisciplinary Team Training Program (www.gittprogram.org/).

REFERENCES

1. Bubshait AA, Farooq G. Team building and project success. *Cost Engineering.* 1999;41:34–38.
2. Gallo JJ, Bogner HR, Fulmer T, Paveza GJ. *Handbook of Geriatric Assessment.* Sudbury, MA: Jones and Bartlett Publishers; 2004.
3. Grumbach K, Bodenheimer T. Can health care teams improve primary care practice? *JAMA.* 2004;291:1246–1251.
4. Moxon P. *Building a Better Team: A Handbook for Managers and Facilitators.* Hants, England: Gower Publishing Co Ltd; 1993.
5. Gordon J. A perspective on team building. *J Am Acad Business.* 2002;2:185–188.
6. Starfield B. *Primary Care.* New York, NY: Oxford University Press; 1998.

CHAPTER | TWELVE

Geriatric Principles

Jeffrey Mariano, MD
Sonja Rosen, MD

MRS BLEWITT'S EXPERIENCE

Mrs Blewitt is seeing you for the first time today. She is 86 years old and just moved from another state to be closer to her son. She lives in a residential care facility and is starting to make new friends. She is healthy, walks every day, and has learned the streets of your town well enough to drive to the market and the symphony. She lost her husband about 5 years ago and has taken Citalopram since then, with good relief of depressive symptoms (she has attempted a taper twice, but had recurrence of depression). Her son is attentive and caring, and he has already helped Mrs Blewitt find bridge games at the local senior center and connected her with the local library to do some reading in their children's program.

INTRODUCTION

Americans have had an increase in life expectancy from 47.3 years in 1900 to 77.2 years in 2000.[1] With longer life expectancy comes an increased likelihood of chronic medical conditions and functional dependence. Older people also suffer from common geriatric syndromes, including cognitive impairment, depression, decreased vision and hearing, incontinence, untreated pain, falls, and social isolation. This chapter provides a brief review of health care maintenance appropriate for older adults and office management of the most common geriatric syndromes.

HEALTH CARE MAINTENANCE AND PREVENTION

Primary prevention is important to help older persons maintain their health and vitality, and includes the following:

➤ *Immunizations:* These should include seasonal influenza annually for patients older than 65, pneumococcal vaccine once for those older than 65, herpes zoster vaccine once for those older than 60, and tetanus every 10 years. Staff can determine immunization status from a previsit questionnaire and should administer needed routine vaccines if no contraindications are identified.

➤ *Exercise:* Aerobic, resistance, and balance exercises are recommended to reduce the risk of heart disease, stroke, and falls. Patients with physical disabilities or limited exercise tolerance can be encouraged to explore different types of exercise programs, such as tai chi or water aerobics.

➤ *Diet:* A diet low in saturated fat and high in fruits, vegetables, and whole grains, and limited alcohol, is recommended.

➤ *Smoking cessation:* Older persons should be educated that smoking cessation at *any* age can lead to improved lung function and decreased mortality.

➤ *Driving assessment:* Car accidents are the leading cause of fatal injury in adults up to age 75, and crash rates for older drivers are higher than any other group except those younger than 25.[1] Physicians should remind patients to wear a seat belt, not drink before driving, obtain necessary aids for sensory impairments, and consider a driving test if there is any concern about the patient's ability to drive safely.

Secondary prevention should take into account the patient's age and life expectancy, functional status, and risks vs benefits of screening.

➤ Women with a remaining life expectancy greater than 5 years should be offered a screening mammogram, given that age alone is the single most important risk factor for women to develop breast cancer.

➤ Screening colonoscopy is recommended every 10 years if normal until age 85.

➤ Prostate specific antigen screening is still controversial for men up to 75 years and is not recommended for men older than 75.

➤ Women older than 65 and men older than 80 should receive osteoporosis screening with a bone mineral density scan.

➤ Men aged 65 to 75 who have ever smoked or have hypertension should receive abdominal aortic aneurysm screening with an abdominal ultrasound.

➤ Dyslipidemia screening is recommended for men and women every 5 years if they do not have coronary artery disease, diabetes mellitus, peripheral artery disease, or stroke, although there are no good data supporting the use of statins as primary prevention in the elderly.

FUNCTIONAL ASSESSMENT

➤ When making health care decisions, utilizing functional age rather than chronologic age is much more appropriate for older adults who are healthy and active.

➤ Functional status is measured by activities of daily living (basic, instrumental, and advanced) and is a useful framework to anticipate care in older adults.

➤ Basic activities of daily living include the ability to bathe, dress, feed, transfer, toilet, and ambulate independently.

➤ Instrumental activities of daily living include the ability to go shopping, prepare food, take medications, use transportation, manage finances, and use the telephone.

➤ Advanced activities of daily living include the ability to fulfill societal, community, and family roles as well as participate in recreational or occupational tasks. These advanced activities vary considerably from individual to individual but may be valuable in monitoring functional status before the development of disability.

➤ In addition, screening for impairments in cognition, vision and hearing, gait, continence, and depression (see below) must be part of the initial examination. These can be carried out by nursing personnel or other members of the team/office staff rather than by the clinician (see the previsit questionnaire on UCLA's Geronet[2]).

➤ Changes in functional status may indicate a new acute medical problem, worsening of a chronic medical condition, medication side effects, or the need for increased caregiver support or transition to a higher level of care.

➤ Poor functional status (ie, impairments in basic activities of daily living) implies underlying medical, cognitive, or psychosocial comorbidities that increase risk of hospitalization, delirium, and death, and delays recovery from acute illness.

➤ A self-administered or staff-administered checklist should be part of the health record (see the previsit questionnaire[2]).

➤ Once decline is documented, community resources such as Meals on Wheels, government-sponsored in-home support, or other community resources can be mobilized.

FALLS/GAIT AND BALANCE

➤ Gait disorders are common in older adults and are a predictor of functional decline. Complications resulting from falls are the leading cause of death from injury in men and women aged 65 and older. More than 500,000 hip fractures occur in the United States annually.[3, 4]

➤ Screening for falls should include asking the question, "Have you fallen in the last 12 months?" and performance of the Timed Get Up and Go test. These tasks can be delegated to staff.

➤ The cause of gait impairment in older adults is usually multifactorial; a full assessment must therefore consider a number of different causes, as determined from a detailed physical examination and gait evaluation.

➤ The causes of a fall often involve a complex interaction among factors intrinsic to the individual (age-related decline, chronic disease, acute illness, medications), challenges to postural control (environment, changing position, normal activities), and mediating factors (risk-taking behaviors, underlying mobility level).

➤ Previsit questionnaires or staff members should routinely ask whether a patient has had a fall; if so, circumstance of the fall should be obtained, including the activity of the faller at the time of the incident, the occurrence of prodromal symptoms (lightheadedness, imbalance, and dizziness), the location of the fall, and the time of the fall.

➤ On the basis of these findings, the appropriate falls intervention can be initiated; this could include outpatient physical therapy, occupational therapy, and a home safety evaluation, as well as referral to community exercise and balance classes.

POLYPHARMACY AND ADVERSE DRUG EVENTS

➤ Age-associated changes in body composition, metabolism, and pharmacody-namics make drug-drug and drug-disease interactions a significant problem for older adults, leading to delirium, falls, and other adverse outcomes.

➤ Risk factors associated with inappropriate prescribing, overprescribing, and underprescribing include having more than one prescriber, poor record keeping, renal insufficiency, and the use of more than one pharmacy.

➤ Cardiovascular drugs, anticoagulants, diuretics, nonsteroidal anti-inflammatory drugs (NSAIDs), hypoglycemics, and atypical antipsychotics are the drug classes most often associated with preventable adverse drug events.

➤ Patients should bring all their medication, including over-the-counter medications, to each appointment. Staff should review them and highlight any changes before the nurse or physician visit.

 ➤ Over-the-counter medications, vitamins, and other herbal supplements purchased at health food stores can lead to drug-drug, drug-age, or drug-disease interactions and should always be included in the patient's medication list and reviewed at each visit.

➤ When a patient develops a new problem, always consider whether it could be due to a medication side effect.

PAIN

➤ Pain should be monitored as the "fifth vital sign." It is also valuable to have staff assess its impact on quality of life.

➤ More than half of older adults suffer from some type of chronic pain, which can lead to functional decline, depression, insomnia, and social withdrawal.

➤ Common causes include degenerative arthritis, neuropathy (diabetic, herpetic, idiopathic), and low-back pain (often due to lumbar stenosis).

➤ Pain should be routinely evaluated to clarify its impact on functional status, sleep, mobility, and mood.

➤ Effective pain management should include appropriate pharmacologic and nonpharmacologic (physical therapy, acupuncture) strategies. An American Geriatrics Society position statement on pain encourages providers to avoid NSAIDs when possible in older adults because of increased risk.[5] Low-dose narcotics can be safe and effective in older adults but should be initiated with a full discussion of risks (confusion, falls, etc) and an appropriate bowel regimen.

➤ If patients older than 75 are prescribed long-term NSAIDs, the Agency for Healthcare Research and Quality Effective Clinical Practice Guidelines recommends a proton pump inhibitor or misoprostol.

URINARY INCONTINENCE

➤ Urinary incontinence (UI) is common among older women and men but often underreported. In fact, many women may think it is a normal part of aging and may also be embarrassed to discuss this problem.

➤ Untreated, UI is associated with depressive symptoms in older persons, in whom it is also a marker of increased risk of mortality.

➤ It is critical that clinicians screen for this common problem in all older patients.

➤ Staff can ask two questions to screen for incontinence: (1) In the last year, have you ever lost your urine or gotten wet? And if so, (2) Have you lost urine on at least six separate days? A positive answer is very sensitive for UI in both men and women. A positive answer can also prompt staff to perform a basic workup for causes of UI, including urinalysis and urine culture to rule out infection and postvoid residual bladder scan or straight catheterization to rule out urinary retention.

➤ Positive culture and/or excessive urinary retention will then guide further workup and treatment.

MALNUTRITION/WEIGHT LOSS

➤ Malnutrition increases the risk of infection, fractures, functional impairment, and mortality.

➤ Previsit questionnaires or staff members should ask patients about unintentional weight loss within the previous 6 months, as weight loss of 10% or more of total body weight over 6 months is concerning. Body mass index (BMI) should be measured; a BMI less than 22 raises the concern of malnutrition.

➤ If a patient has abnormal weight loss, the clinician needs to determine whether this is secondary to undereating or a catabolic process.

➤ If a patient is under-eating, causes can include lack of access to food, dental or other oral health issues, depression, underlying cognitive impairment, or functional impairments making food preparation difficult.

DEPRESSION

➤ Older adults have significant losses and changes in health that they are unable to regulate; as a result, it is common for them to have a depressed mood and potentially be diagnosed with depression.

➤ Older adults may present with atypical symptoms of depression, including somatization. Challenges in symptom recognition occur with comorbid medical or cognitive disorders.

➤ The single screening question, "Do you often feel sad or depressed?" may miss some older patients with depression. Therefore, it is best used in conjunction with other screening tests, such as the Geriatric Depression Scale or the Patient Health Questionnaire-9 (PHQ-9). The latter is a self-administered survey that staff can give to patients to complete before the visit with the physician.

➤ Older adults may have some preconceived negative ideas about depression. As a result, it is important to help them understand that they can get help with their feelings and symptoms (eg, sleep, appetite). Both talk therapy and pharmacologic therapy have been proven effective. Helping patients understand the opportunities to help them cope with their losses is important and should be done on a regular basis.

COGNITIVE IMPAIRMENT

➤ The prevalence of cognitive impairment, including mild cognitive impairment, Alzheimer disease, vascular dementias, and other dementias increases with age.

➤ There are several validated, physician-administered tools to screen for cognitive impairment. These include the Mini-Mental State Examination (proprietary), the Saint Louis University Mental Status Examination, and the Montreal Cognitive Assessment, as well as shorter screens such as the Mini-Cog test, which combines three-item recall and the clock-draw test.

➤ Staff are often an integral part of care of cognitively impaired patients. They can help coordinate the patients' care with other subspecialists and between disciplines and, often most importantly, work with families. Input from a social worker, if available, is invaluable to the care of patients with cognitive impairment.

SENSORY IMPAIRMENT

Vision Impairment

➤ Vision impairment increases in prevalence with age and is most commonly due to cataracts. Age-related macular degeneration, diabetic retinopathy, and glaucoma must also be considered.

➤ As vision impairment is associated with increased risk of falls and overall decreased functional status, its detection and treatment are most important.

➤ Staff can administer the Snellen eye chart to screen for vision impairment.

Hearing Impairment

➤ Hearing impairment affects approximately one-third of persons older than 65 and is associated with reduced cognitive, physical, and social function.[6, 7]

➤ The simplest screening test is to rely on the patient's own subjective report of hearing loss. Staff can ask patients whether they feel they have hearing impairment, and an affirmative answer is a positive test for hearing loss.

➤ The whisper test is another good screening test, which staff can also be trained to administer.

➤ An audioscope can also be used to objectively test for hearing loss.

➤ Any patient with hearing impairment should be referred to an audiologist.

ADVANCE CARE PLANNING

Four guiding ethical principles of American medical practice are beneficence, nonmaleficence, justice, and respect for autonomy. It is often helpful for the clinician to explore a patient's hopes and fears and to help the patient clarify his or her goals so that treatment options are based on these goals.

➤ Assigning a Durable Power of Attorney for Health Care is an important first step to obtaining substituted judgment.

➤ Patients should also complete an Advance Directive to outline their wishes.

➤ Some states have implemented a Physician Orders for Life Sustaining Treatment Program to translate advance directives into physician orders to ensure that a patient's wishes are followed.

➤ Using functional outcomes as a means to frame future treatments may be helpful. For example, patients may be asked, "If the doctors could do these life-sustaining procedures to prolong your life but you were still unable to do that special activity [ie, feeding] you mentioned, would you want that procedure to be done?"

➤ This information should be kept in a prominent place in the medical record for use by the health care team and family.

The importance of a full, appropriately detailed physical examination, with emphasis on functional status, cannot be overstated. As this generation of geriatric patients ages, it is important to acknowledge the functional, medical, and psychosocial heterogeneity that exists. However, because of their medical and cognitive conditions, many older adults are unable to accurately report symptoms. The clinician cannot assume that "no news is good news" in the care of older adults. By being aware of these geriatric principles, and by empowering and educating the staff to assist in geriatric assessment, a stronger, more proactive team can be mobilized on the patient's behalf to maintain wellness and independent functioning.

USEFUL RESOURCES

Ganz DA, Bao Y, Shekelle PG, et al. Will my patient fall? *JAMA*. 2007;297(1):77–86.

Fick DM, Cooper JW, Wade WE, et al. Updating the Beers criteria for potentially inappropriate medication use in older adults: results of a US consensus panel of experts. *Arch Intern Med*. 2003;163(22):2716–2724.

Fleming KC, Evans JM. Practical functional assessment of elderly persons: a primary-care approach. *Mayo Clin Proc*. 1995;70(9):890–910.

Rosen S, Reuben DB. Principles of geriatric assessment. In: Halter JB, Ouslander JG, Tinetti ME, et al, eds. *Hazzard's Geriatric Medicine and Gerontology*. 6th ed. New York, NY: McGraw-Hill Inc; 2009.

Reuben DB, Herr KA, Pacula JT, et al. *Geriatrics at Your Fingertips: 2008–2009*. 10th ed. New York, NY: American Geriatrics Society; 2008 (https://fulfillment.frycomm.com/ags/gayf/order_form.asp for the form, or http://www.americangeriatrics.org/publications/shop_publications/ for publications page).

Geriatric Screening Tools

➤ Mini-Cog: http://geriatrics.uthscsa.edu/tools/MINICog.pdf.

➤ Saint Louis University Mental Status Examination: http://medschool.slu.edu/agingsuccessfully/pdfsurveys/slumsexam_05.pdf.

➤ Montreal Cognitive Assessment: www.mocatest.org/pdf_files/MoCA-Test-English.pdf.

➤ Timed Get Up and Go Test: www.hospitalmedicine.org/geriresource/toolbox/pdfs/get_up_and_go_test.pdf.

➤ Personal Health Questionnaire Depression Scale (PHQ-9): http://patienteducation.stanford.edu/research/phq.pdf.

➤ Geriatric Depression Scale: www.mhsfopcls.com/downloads/ger_dep_scl.pdf.

➤ Activities of Daily Living/Independent Activities of Daily Living: www.mhsfopcls.com/downloads/ger_dep_scl.pdf.

➤ Measuring medical care provided to vulnerable elders: the Assessing Care of Vulnerable Elders-3 (ACOVE 3) Quality Indicators. *JAGS*. 2007:55(suppl 2):S247–S487.

➤ US Preventive Services Task Force Guide to Clinical Preventive Services. http://www.ahrq.gov/clinic/cps3dix.htm

➤ American Geriatrics Society. Geriatrics Review Syllabus. https://fulfillment.frycomm.com/ags/grs7_order_form.asp

REFERENCES

1. Centers for Disease Control and Prevention. *United States Life Tables, 2000*. National Vital Statistics Reports. Atlanta, GA: U.S. Department of Health and Human Services, Centers for Disease Control and Prevention. Available at: http://www.cdc.gov/nchs/data/nvsr/nvsr51/nvsr51_03.pdf

2. UCLA Previsit Questionnaire. www.geronet.ucla.edu/centers/acove/office_forms.htm.

3. Centers for Disease Control and Prevention. *Hip fractures Among Older Adults*. Atlanta, GA: U.S. Department of Health and Human Services, Centers for Disease Control and Prevention; 2002. Available at: http://www.cdc.gov/ncipc/factsheets/adulthipfx.htm#how%20big%20is%20problem

4. Ganz DA, Bao Y, Shekelle PF, et al. Will my patient fall? *JAMA*. 2007;297(1):77–86.

5. American Geriatrics Society Clinical Practice Guideline: Pharmacological Management of Persistent Pain in Older Persons. http://www.ahrq.gov/clinic/cps3dix.htm

6. National Institutes of Health, National Institute on Deafness and Other Communication Disorders Web site. Accessed at http://www.nidcd.nih.gov/health/statistics/quick.htm.

7. Dalton SD, Cruickshanks KJ, Klein BE, et al. "The impact of hearing loss on quality of life in older adults." The Gerontologist. 2003:43(5):661–668. http://www.clas.ufl.edu/users/mcolburn/Web-links/SPA4321/Impact%20of%20HL%20on%20QOL.pdf

CHAPTER THIRTEEN

Geriatric-Friendly Forms

Grace Chen, MD

David B. Reuben, MD

MRS BLEWITT'S EXPERIENCE

In your first visit with Mrs Blewitt, the medical assistant reviews her previsit questionnaire with her and determines that Mrs Blewitt has not had a tetanus shot in many years, does not think she has ever had a pneumococcal vaccine, and has never heard of the shingles vaccine. She reports that Mrs Blewitt remembered two of three items on the Mini-Cog but did not plan well enough on her clock and could not fit an "11" on the face. Mrs Blewitt had to use her hands to stand on the Get Up and Go test but could complete the test in 9 seconds. Mrs Blewitt failed the whisper test, which prompted your assistant to check for earwax and have the patient's ears cleaned before you even entered the room. The assistant placed a Saint Louis University Mental Status Examination on the chart for you to complete and initiated a physical therapy consultation for gait and balance evaluation, pending your approval. She asked you to discuss the shingles vaccine and promised to have the other vaccines ready by the time you had completed your examination. She also provided Mrs Blewitt with a list of adult day health care centers in the area, as Mrs Blewitt had asked for ways to stay active.

INTRODUCTION

Forms filled out by the patient in preparation for the visit with the physician can help make the visit more efficient and goal directed. Likewise, standardized forms for common chronic syndromes facilitate tracking of progress and treatment.

PREVISIT QUESTIONNAIRE

Initial Visit

Many new patients older than 64 who present for an initial assessment have an extensive medical and social history, so it is helpful to gather as much of this information as possible before the appointment. The initial visit gathers information to direct evaluation of medical conditions, initiate treatment plans, and mobilize resources. If a patient has cognitive impairment, a previsit form completed by a caregiver is invaluable. A sample of the form can be accessed at www.geronet.ucla.edu/centers/acove/office_forms.htm.

A previsit questionnaire is most effective when it accomplishes the following goals: (1) facilitates information collection, (2) directs the visit to focus on the most pressing issues, (3) identifies key geriatric syndromes and issues, and (4) facilitates documentation.

It should:

➤ Be comprehensive but not overly cumbersome (to increase likelihood of form completion)

➤ Avoid medical jargon

➤ Give specific choices rather than open-ended questions

➤ Address the most common problems that affect older populations

➤ Address geriatric syndromes

➤ Include functional assessment

➤ Avoid inclusion of too many items that are helpful in research but yield little clinical relevance

➤ Allow the information to be easily transferrable to the electronic medical record

The initial visit previsit questionnaire should contain the following:

➤ Demographic information (including who filled out the form and contact information)

➤ Traditional aspects of the medical history

    ➤ Past medical history

        ➤ Include most common/frequent medical conditions by system

    ➤ Past surgical history

    ➤ Hospitalizations in last 5 years

    ➤ Allergies

        ➤ Include description of reactions

➤ Medications

    ➤ List of medications with their doses and frequencies

    ➤ Include prescriptions, over-the-counter products, and supplements

    ➤ Assess for method of taking medications

➤ Social history, including:

    ➤ Living situation, including what type of home, with whom patient lives, and any recent changes

    ➤ Marital status

    ➤ Education level

    ➤ Previous occupation(s)

    ➤ Contact information of family/friends

    ➤ Type and extent of help from family members and/or employed help

    ➤ Alcohol screening

    ➤ Tobacco screening

    ➤ Illicit drug use screening

    ➤ Domestic violence screening

➤ Family history

➤ Functional assessment

    ➤ Level of independence with basic and instrumental activities of daily living

    ➤ Driving status

    ➤ Who provides assistance, if needed

➤ Advance directives

    ➤ Assess for durable medical power of attorney

    ➤ Assess for living will, physician orders for life-sustaining treatment (if relevant; www.polst.org), and advance directives and confirm wishes

➤ Health maintenance

    ➤ Vaccinations

    ➤ Age-appropriate screening measures and relevant results

    ➤ Most recent dental, vision, and hearing examinations

➤ Review of systems for past 3 months

    ➤ By system

➤ Personal Health Questionnaire two-question screen for depression

➤ Fall assessment

The previsit questionnaire is successful only if it is completed before the initial visit. The most common challenges to form completion are lack of access (such as not receiving the form in a timely manner before the appointment), poor health literacy, and language barriers. Mechanisms should be in place for the patient or patient surrogate to have access to the forms before the visit. If an electronic medical record is available, the form should be accessible through a portal for the patient to complete before the visit. In addition, the data entered by the patient and/or surrogate should prepopulate the clinician's notes to increase efficiency. For practices that do not have electronic medical records or patients who do not have Internet access, the form should be sent by mail for the patient to complete or be sent by e-mail to a surrogate. If there is inadequate time for the postal service to deliver the questionnaire or there is no e-mail, the patient can be instructed to arrive 30 minutes early to fill out the form. Likewise, if the patient has a literacy (due to lack of education or visual impairment) or language barrier, the form should be completed by a surrogate who can understand the form.

Follow-Up Visits

A previsit questionnaire completed by the patient and/or surrogate before follow-up visits helps focus the visit on the most pressing issues for the patient and updates the physician on interval changes since the last visit. For example, patients are asked to list the two most important issues they wish to address with the physician and are also screened for falls, incontinence, and weight loss. In addition, visits to other physicians and an updated medications list, including request for refills, are assessed. A prompt for the patient to list contact information for the pharmacy expedites the refill process.

Focused-Problem Visit Forms

As a result of the Assessing Care of Vulnerable Elders (ACOVE) studies, structured visit initial and follow-up notes on the topics of depression, heart failure, falls, urinary incontinence, and dementia have been developed.[1] These forms can help guide office visits on these conditions and facilitate tracking of progress on these chronic issues and treatment. These forms also provide in-depth history, physical examination, and treatment options/guides. The subjective section is typically set up in such a way that the information can be prepopulated by the nurse or office assistant when the patient is being placed into the rooms and/or having vital signs assessed. Similarly, some simple assessment tasks (eg, orthostatic vital signs, vision testing) can be assessed by staff and prepopulated in the notes. All of these forms can be accessed at www.geronet.ucla.edu/centers/acove/office_forms.htm.

USEFUL RESOURCES

UCLA Geronet: Health & Aging Resources for Higher Education. Office forms for healthcare professionals (www.geronet.ucla.edu/centers/acove/office_forms.htm).

Personal Health Questionnaire two-question depression screen (PHQ-2) (http://health.utah.gov/mihp/pdf/PHQ-9%20two%20question.pdf).

REFERENCE

1. Assessing Care of Vulnerable Elders (ACOVE): a Rand Health Project. www.rand.org/health/projects/acove/. Accessed December 3, 2009.

CHAPTER FOURTEEN

Visit Flow: Enhancing the Experience for Patients and Clinicians

Allison Lindauer, FNP, GNP

MRS BLEWITT'S EXPERIENCE

At your last visit with Mrs Blewitt you identified mild cognitive impairment and worked with her son to have him set up a weekly medication box for her through her assisted living facility. You identified poor hearing, and she has seen an audiologist; Mrs Blewitt now has new hearing aids. Her immunization record was updated by your staff, and she has seen a physical therapist to work on gait and balance. Today she comes back complaining of worsening urinary incontinence. Your staff had her fill out the previsit questionnaire and placed her in a room with an electric table in case you need to do a pelvic examination. A urinalysis has been done and is positive for leukocytes and nitrites.

INTRODUCTION

Providers who see older patients are intimately familiar with the need to maximize efficiency during ambulatory visits. This chapter reviews tips to tailor clinical flow to the needs of the patient, the family, and the clinician to help make visits both productive and meaningful.

VISIT FLOW

For many of our geriatric patients, medical care early in their lives consisted of a physician providing one-on-one care for a patient in the patient's home. As our patients aged, medical care transformed into a sophisticated process carried out mostly in offices. For our patients, care now involves traveling to an office and interacting with many people (including front office staff, medical assistants, nurses, and ancillary professionals) in concert with complex technology. Providing care for our older patients necessitates an appreciation of their history combined with a respect for the physical challenges many elders have.

Practices that embrace the skills of all staff allow for the care and support of each patient, while at the same time respecting the pressures placed on the modern clinician. Office flow patterns that employ the talents of all involved allow for parallel care. Parallel care maximizes clinician time by allowing other professionals to provide services to a patient while the clinician is caring for a separate patient.[1]

Mrs Blewitt's experience illustrates this pattern of parallel care. While the clinician is with another patient, office personnel take the initiative to assist Mrs Blewitt in filling out questionnaires. The medical staff evaluates concerns and procures a urine sample before the clinician visit. Mrs Blewitt is placed in a room that accommodates her needs (an electric table is in the room). Teams that function well provide the clinician with "found time": time to practice the caring arts without feeling beleaguered by instructing staff in each step of care.

The beauty of geriatric care is that there are many opportunities to allow professional staff to accept ownership of their role in care. Making the office visit for the older patient comfortable is a complex process that demands the input of many workers over time. Box 14-1 features a list of steps and practices that help ensure your patient has a positive practice experience.

MRS BLEWITT'S FOLLOW-UP

You discuss with Mrs Blewitt that her incontinence is likely from a urinary tract infection, and you prescribe a course of antibiotics. A pelvic examination shows poor perineal tone, so you send her to physical therapy for incontinence exercises. You print two copies of your after-visit summary and request that her son keep one copy so that he can help monitor for any symptoms of urinary tract complications.

Box 14-1 Checklist of Older-Adult-Friendly Practice Tips

Preparation to see provider

1. *Arrival:* Ensure wheelchair accessibility. Include answers to common transportation questions (eg, parking options such as valet, garage, parking lot; nearest subway/bus stations) with the appointment reminder or previsit questionnaire.

2. *Check-in:* Train the front office staff to be sensitive to memory and hearing issues.

3. *Medical assistant's role:* A trained medical assistant can assist by completing the following:

   ➤ Medication review

      ➤ Include the patient and family in understanding the medication list. Review the Medication Administration Record (MAR) if patient lives in a facility. Coach the family to bring the MAR, and ask the medical assistant to call to have it faxed if the patient arrives without it.

      ➤ Print out the medication list, record changes since the last visit.

      ➤ List all over the counter medicines (OTC's) on the medication list.

      ➤ Ensure long-term, stable medications are filled as a 3-month supply with a year's worth of refills (or as maximally allowed on the patient's medication plan).

      ➤ Record a consistent pharmacy (both mail order and local).

   ➤ Vital signs. Include orthostatics once a year or as clinically indicated; weight; body mass index; evaluation for 10% weight loss in the last year; hearing and vision screen

   ➤ Evaluation for critical events (falls, food insecurity, transportation issues)

   ➤ Updating of social history (allows for bond between provider and patient). Add key element to "break the ice" (eg "I remember your story about delivering mail in rural Oregon.")

   ➤ Other testing as appropriate, such as checking for ear wax, checking nails, and performing the Get Up and Go test, Mini-Cog, and/or geriatric depression scale.

Provider Visit: History

1. Introduce yourself every single time (this protects dignity for patients with cognitive impairment).

2. Make sure the patient is comfortable and can hear you (the medical assistant should remind you if you need to use a "pocket talker," a portable voice amplification device).

3. Elicit patient concerns and negotiate an agenda for the visit that balances the patient concerns with your concerns (eg, the patient with dementia may worry more about something "irrelevant"). Acknowledging her concern promotes her dignity ("I hear that you are very worried about your cat; I'm sorry to see you so concerned"). This reduces patient's anxiety and can facilitate flow.

4. Address clinician concerns

   ➤ Review inappropriate medications, update medication list, confirm long-term medicines

   ➤ Evaluate for geriatric syndromes

(continued)

Box 14-1 (continued)

- Evaluate for critical events (falls, confusion, incontinence, weight loss)
- Assess social concerns such as financial issues, driving, education level, and caregiver strain
- Evaluate lifestyle factors such as tobacco, alcohol, and exercise
- Prioritize and evaluate need for preventive care. Preventive counseling includes a discussion about when to "graduate" from screening (ie, screening is no longer indicated).

Provider Visit: Physical Examination

Much of the physical examination can occur with pure observation while you interview the patient (eg, evaluate gait as she walks to the room). Geriatric patients often require the following:

1. Check teeth and mouth for pain, loose dentures, and lesions that could be malignant.
2. Check skin for actinic keratoses or other premalignant or malignant lesions.
3. Check feet to evaluate whether nails need trimming.
4. Screen for geriatric syndromes:
   - Mini-Cog: http://geriatrics.uthscsa.edu/tools/MINICog.pdf
   - Saint Louis University Mental Status Examination: http://medschool.slu.edu/agingsuccessfully/pdfsurveys/slumsexam_05.pdf
   - Timed Get Up and Go Test: www.hospitalmedicine.org/geriresource/toolbox/pdfs/get_up_and_go_test.pdf
   - Personal Health Questionnaire Depression Scale (PHQ-9): http://patienteducation.stanford.edu/research/phq.pdf
   - Geriatric Depression Scale: www.mhsfopcls.com/downloads/ger_dep_scl.pdf
   - Activities of Daily Living/ Independent Activities of Daily Living: http://webmedia.unmc.edu/intmed/geriatrics/reynolds/pearlcards/functionaldisability/activities_of_daily_living.htm
5. Perform other examination elements as indicated.
6. Prescribe appropriate medications, laboratory work, and therapies as indicated.
7. Enlist external services as indicated (eg, Meals on Wheels, Home Care, Housing Consultant).
8. Assist the patient with forms as needed.
   - Advance directives
   - Family Medical Leave Act
   - Department of Motor Vehicle forms: handicapped permit, impaired driver

Fostering Communication for Patients in Facilities

1. If the patient lives in an institutional facility, and you have an electronic medical record, it is often worthwhile to take a few extra minutes to finish your note so you can send a copy back to the facility.
2. Call the facility with any questions.

3. Have a speaker phone available in the room so you can use it to call facility staff if needed.

4. Ask the facility to send written information with each visit (what are their concerns?).

After-Visit Summary

You should standardize an after-visit summary for all your patients that includes:

➤ Vital signs, name of provider, telephone number, medication list

➤ Written instructions for any changes to medications and lifestyle changes you recommend

➤ Individualized patient goals

Print out the after-visit summary in large font (eg, 16 pt) and give it to the patient to take home.

REFERENCE

1. Ganz DA, Fung CH, Sinsky CA, et al. Key elements of high-quality primary care for vulnerable elders. *J Gen Intern Med.* 2008;23(12):2018–2023.

CHAPTER FIFTEEN

Billing Opportunities

Audrey Chun, MD

MRS BLEWITT'S EXPERIENCE

Mrs Blewitt does well under your care for another year, but then is hospitalized with another urinary tract infection, this time complicated by delirium and several falls. Fortunately, she does not break any bones (thanks to your good care of her osteoporosis). She is discharged back to her residential care facility, but her son calls you panicked the next day because she is disheveled and not speaking clearly and has fallen again. Your staff has given the patient an urgent slot just before the noon break and has notified your social worker that she will need to participate in the visit. The social worker has already called the facility to learn more about their levels of care and found that they have an assisted living wing that has an opening. The facility has faxed the admit orders so they are available when the patient arrives. You and the social worker spend 75 minutes in a family conference with the patient and son, including completing all the orders for her move to assisted living. You explain to the son the lasting effects delirium can have and outline additional care needs Mrs Blewitt has now. You place an order for home health, and 2 days later you review the home care plan and sign off on the certification.

INTRODUCTION

One challenge of geriatric care can be adequate reimbursement for the time spent on caring for patients who may require intensive care coordination, family meetings to address goals of care, and extra time for appropriate disease management and education. However, practitioners often do not recognize that there are opportunities for billing and reimbursement to get credit for the care they are providing.

Because most older adults are covered by Medicare, this discussion focuses on billing opportunities within the Center for Medicare and Medicaid Services (CMS) guidelines that are in addition to the evaluation/management (E/M) services with which most providers are familiar. The Current Procedural Terminology (CPT®) codes are specific for the outpatient/ambulatory setting and are distinct from those codes associated with skilled nursing facilities or hospice, although conceptually there will be similarities in requirements and documentation for services provided. This chapter will focus on billing for prolonged services within a visit, home care certification/recertification, and care plan oversight.

E/M SERVICES

CPT Codes

➤ New patient: 99201-99205

➤ Established patient: 99211-99215

➤ Remember that for visits where more than 50% of the visit was spent in *face-to-face* counseling and/or care coordination, you may bill according to the time spent with the patient. This generally works best for follow-up visits; time requirements are summarized in Table 15-1.[1]

➤ For detailed requirements for each level of billing and component of documentation, please refer to the CMS E/M guide.[1]

TABLE 15-1 E/M Coding When >50% Is Spent in Counseling and/or Care Coordination

Appropriate E/M Code	Total Length of Visit (min)
99211	5
99212	10
99213	15
99214	25
99215	40

PROLONGED SERVICES

Prolonged service codes should be used in a setting when more than an hour is spent on services for a patient in addition to what would be expected for the E/M code billed. Box 15-1 outlines the requirements necessary to bill for prolonged services.[2,3]

CPT Codes

➤ 99354: Both the E/M code and code 99354 should be submitted for the date of service. Code 99354 can be used only once per encounter regardless of the amount of time spent with the patient. Note that despite the language in the description, there are threshold times when you can begin billing for the prolonged service codes; these are described in Table 15-2.

➤ 99355: Each 30-minute unit, greater than the one unit of code 99354, can be added multiple times to the charge, as appropriate for each 30-minute interval. Table 15-2 lists the threshold times for billing code 99355, which would be in addition to the E/M code and one unit of code 99354.

Examples of Covered Services

➤ In the case of Mrs Blewitt, she is seen for follow-up of medical issues from a recent hospitalization as well as extensive care coordination related to her transition to an assisted living facility. Total face-to-face time was 75 minutes. You can bill code 99215 based on having spent greater than 50% time of at least 40 minutes in counseling and coordination of care.

Box 15-1 Requirements for Prolonged Services Billing

Must be face to face and billed in addition to an E/M code on same date.

Documentation must show:

➤ Medical justification for prolonged services

➤ Sufficient evidence that services were face to face

➤ Start and stop times

➤ Date of service

TABLE 15-2 Threshold Times for Prolonged Visit Codes

E/M Code	Typical Time for E/M Code (min)	Threshold Time to Bill Code 99354 (min)	Threshold Time to Bill Codes 99354+99355 (min)
99201	10	40	85
99202	20	50	95
99203	30	60	105
99204	45	75	120
99205	60	90	135
99212	10	40	85
99213	15	45	90
99214	25	55	100
99215	40	70	115

Because the total face-to-face time meets the threshold for prolonged services of the E/M code 99215 (70 minutes), an additional *one* unit of code 99354 can be billed concomitantly.

➤ A patient sees you for diabetes and recently diagnosed metastatic colon cancer, during which extensive counseling and discussion of goals of care/advance directives occurs. The patient's daughter arrives midway through the visit and has some concerns about her father's decisions that required additional counseling and exploration of the patient's goals and how they might relate to the daughter's concerns. Total face-to-face time is 120 minutes. You can bill code 99215 based on having spent greater than 50% time of at least 40 minutes in counseling and coordination of care. Because the total face-to-face time meets the threshold for prolonged services beyond the E/M code 99215, an additional *one* unit of code 99354 can be billed concomitantly with an additional *one* unit of code 99355 for 30 minutes of additional service by meeting the threshold of at least 115 minutes.

Example of Service Not Covered

➤ A patient was in the office for 1 hour receiving nebulizer treatment for mild asthma exacerbation meeting criteria for E/M code 99213, but face-to-face time with the billing provider was only 20 minutes (face-to-face time of more than 45 minutes would have been required to meet the threshold time to bill for prolonged services code 99354).

> ### Box 15-2 Requirements for Billing Home Care Certification/Recertification
>
> Documentation must show:
>
> ➤ Patient is homebound and requires skilled services (include diagnosis)
>
> ➤ Plan of care is established and reviewed by billing provider
>
> ➤ Service is provided while under care of the billing provider
>
> For recertification:
>
> ➤ All of the above, and
>
> > ➤ Obtained at time of review of plan of care
> >
> > ➤ Continued need for skilled care per initial certification

HOME CARE BILLING

➤ Home care certification and recertification codes should be used for initiation or recertification of home care services in conjunction with the plan of care for patients receiving Medicare-covered home services. There is no time requirement for these services (see Box 15-2). These should not be billed when Medicaid or private insurance is covering home health services.[4]

HEALTHCARE COMMON PROCEDURE CODING SYSTEM LEVEL II CODES

➤ G0180: certification (no Medicare-covered home care services in last 60 days)

➤ G0179: recertification (once every 60 days)

Examples of Covered Services

➤ A patient sees you for diabetes and an ulcer formed after trauma related to an accidental fall. Wound care, physical therapy, and diabetic education are medically necessary, and you initiate wound care and physical therapy home services with a home health agency that bills Medicare for services provided. You establish and review the plan of care.

Example of Service Not Covered

➤ Same patient as above, but home services are being billed to Medicaid

CARE PLAN OVERSIGHT (CPO)

This covers services related to complex or multidisciplinary care modalities as part of Medicare-covered services by a participating home health agency. Box 15-3 outlines the requirements necessary to bill for CPO. These services do not need to be face to face but must add up to at least 30 minutes of time spent in care plan oversight in a calendar month. See Table 15-3 for a sample template to track CPO minutes.[5,6]

CPT Code

➤ G0181

Examples of Acceptable Care Modalities

➤ Physician development/revision of care plan

➤ Reviewing reports of patient status

Box 15-3 Requirements for CPO Billing

➤ Provider cannot have financial arrangement with or be employed by the home health agency

➤ Only one provider per month may bill CPO for a given patient

➤ Does not count for end-stage renal disease capitation or postsurgery follow-up

➤ Billing provider must be provider who signed the certification for home health services

➤ Face-to-face service within 6 months prior

➤ At least 30 minutes of service in one calendar month

➤ Patient must be receiving Medicare-covered home health during time CPO is billed

➤ Patient must require complex or multidisciplinary care modalities requiring ongoing physician involvement in patient's plan of care

TABLE 15-3 CPO Documentation Sample

Patient:	

MR#/DOB:	

Month:	December 2009

Date	Description	Start Time	End Time	Minutes
12-1	INR reviewed, Coumadin adjusted, and new dose discussed with nurse to change meds in pill box	5:25p	5:30p	5
12-9	Wound with additional drainage - changed wound care orders	4:15p	4:22p	7
12-14	INR reviewed, Coumadin adjusted, and new dose discussed with nurse to change meds in pill box	5:25p	5:30p	5
12-16	Physical therapist called with concerns of elevated BP	10:17a	10:22a	5
12-17	Reviewed BP flowsheet sent by RN	1:45p	1:47p	2
12-17	Spoke with home care nurse regarding BP fluctuation - adjusted medication dose	12:05p	12:10p	5
12-28	INR reviewed, Coumadin adjusted, and new dose discussed with nurse to change meds in pill box	5:30p	5:36p	6
			Total minutes:	35

➤ Review of related labs or other studies (not related to E/M services billed during a face to face visit)

➤ Communication with other providers, not at the same practice as the billing provider

➤ Integration of new information into treatment plan

➤ Adjustment of medical therapy

Examples of Services Not Countable

➤ Time spent traveling

➤ Staff time for filing or getting charts

➤ Renewing prescriptions unless discussion with pharmacist is related to care plan

➤ Time spent speaking with patient, family, and friends to adjust medication or treatment

➤ Discharge services

➤ Informal consultations with physicians not treating the patient

➤ Communication with staff within your own practice

➤ Time spent preparing/submitting claims

A NOTE ABOUT TELEPHONE ENCOUNTERS

Current Medicare guidelines consider payment for telephone calls to be bundled in with the payments it makes for E/M services, except under the provisions of telemedicine (www.cms.hhs.gov/Telemedicine/). However, some insurers will reimburse for telephone communications related to care for non-Medicare patients, and it may be worthwhile to follow up with your most commonly used insurers regarding CPT codes 99371 through 99373 for telephone case management.

USEFUL RESOURCE

➤ CMS manual (www.cms.hhs.gov/Manuals/IOM/list.asp).

   ➤ Fee schedule administration and Coding Requirements: (www.cms.gov/manuals/downloads/clm104c23.pdf).

REFERENCES

1. Medicare Learning Network. Evaluation and Management Services Guide. www.cms.hhs.gov/MLNProducts/downloads/eval_mgmt_serv_guide.pdf.

2. MLN Matters, No. MM5972. April 11, 2008. www.cms.hhs.gov/MLNMattersArticles/downloads/MM5972.pdf.

3. CMS Manual System, publication 100-04 Medicare Claims Processing. April 11, 2008, pp. 7, 9–10. www.cms.hhs.gov/Transmittals/Downloads/R1490CP.pdf.

4. CMS. Medicare General Information, Eligibility, and Entitlement, Chapter 4: Physician Certification and Recertification of Services, p. 10. www.cms.hhs.gov/manuals/downloads/ge101c04.pdf.

5. CMS. Medicare Claims Processing Manual, Chapter 12: Physicians/Nonphysician Practitioners, p. 174. www.cms.hhs.gov/manuals/downloads/clm104c12.pdf.

6. CMS. Medicare Benefit Policy Manual, Chapter 15: Covered Medical and Other Health Services, p. 15. www.cms.hhs.gov/Manuals/downloads/bp102c15.pdf.

CHAPTER SIXTEEN

Managing Scheduling Complexities for Older Patients

Robin Telerant, MD

Debbi Shackelford

Elizabeth Eckstrom, MD, MPH

Scheduling clinic appointments for a geriatric population provides a myriad of challenges. Multidisciplinary care is a cornerstone of geriatric medicine and, as such, the clinic scheduler is a critical member of the health care team. This chapter will focus on the importance of up-to-date medical records, timing of appointments, appointment length, and reduction of no-shows, in addition to other details important to optimal geriatric scheduling.

CLARIFICATION OF MEDICAL RECORDS

A reliable point of contact for each patient is indispensible to schedulers, medical assistants, and physicians alike. While a telephone number and address may suffice for younger patients, older patients often have additional needs. Hearing and vision problems make standard telephone calls and letters unanswerable. Cognitive impairment may lead to forgotten appointments or inability to locate the clinic. For these reasons, an appointed decision maker, family member, or facility representative often participates in communication with health care providers. In some cases, more than one of these parties is involved in a patient's care: one participant may organize a patient's appointment schedule, while another might assist with transportation needs. Awareness of the various roles in a patient's care team is critical to facilitate scheduling appointments and timely arrival at and departure from the clinic. An electronic medical record that has flexibility in the number of additional contacts, with notations regarding different roles, is very useful. In a smaller practice, the scheduler may become familiar with each patient's care network and thus know exactly who to contact; however, in a larger practice this detailed information must be kept up to date in the medical record.

TIMING OF APPOINTMENTS

Attendance at outpatient appointments can be a struggle for many older patients. Mobility issues can make leaving the house a challenging endeavor, and finding suitable transportation may lead to further delays. Thus, scheduling elderly patients in the early morning hours can lead to a high no-show or late arrival rate. However, as the day progresses, patients can become fatigued or even irritable. A scheduler may want to ask patients "Are you a morning person?" or "Do you need additional time to get here?" These simple questions can optimize scheduling of older patients.

Scheduling an urgent appointment can also present difficulties in a busy practice, as patients may need to arrange for a clinic time outside of their comfort zone, and presenting for the next available appointment may not be possible. An understanding of this dynamic, as well as having flexibility in scheduling, can help patients with urgent needs.

Given the challenges inherent in finding the appropriate appointment time in this population, one strategy is to schedule appointments ahead of time throughout the year, at whatever interval is most appropriate (monthly, quarterly, etc). While some clinics use an open-access system of scheduling, this leaves little time for planning around an appointment. Scheduling ahead of time allows family, friends, or the facility involved in the care of the patient to be adequately prepared.

APPOINTMENT LENGTH

Older patients often have multiple chronic conditions. Additionally, hearing trouble and cognitive impairment necessitate longer appointment times. A longer clinic visit ensures higher quality of care. A common practice is to allow 30 minutes for a follow-up appointment and a full hour for an annual checkup or new-patient visit. As many patients have complex medical, social, and psychological needs, revenue can be accrued by billing for counseling time (see Chapter 15: Billing Opportunities).

NO-SHOW AND CANCELLATION PREVENTION

Many clinics have protocols in place to prevent late cancellations and absenteeism. These include reminder phone calls or letters and rules regarding dismissal from clinic after a number of missed appointments. When appointment reminders are sent to an older patient population, calls must be delivered to the appropriate party, as the patient may not be responsible for scheduling and transportation to appointments. Moreover, rules regarding dismissal from a practice might be softened or disregarded entirely in this population. Common reasons for no-shows relate to transportation issues or miscommunication regarding the time or location of the appointment. Additionally, in a chronically ill aging population, visits are often missed when the patient is hospitalized or too ill to leave the home. No-shows can be reduced by clear communication and a staff familiar with transportation options for each patient. Older adults face many challenges to being on time for ambulatory appointments. A scheduling staff that is familiar with the myriad of transportation issues that arise, the many people often involved in orchestrating appointments, and the sheer tumult of making it to an appointment on time will ensure that the majority of older patients are prepared and happy when you walk into the room to see them.

TAKE-HOME POINTS

➤ Document important contact information, including patient, family or surrogate decision maker, and address or facility name.

➤ Optimize appointment times to meet the needs of older patients.

➤ Schedule longer appointment times.

➤ Modify no-show policy to accommodate older patients.

➤ Provide resources for transportation to and from the clinic.

➤ Respect the importance of your clinic scheduler.

CHAPTER | SEVENTEEN

Dealing With Transportation Issues

Diana L. White, PhD

Margaret B. Neal, PhD

PATIENT EXPERIENCES

Transportation is becoming more of an issue for your older patients and for your clinic. What has surprised you is the wide range of needs and issues your patients face. In the past 2 weeks alone, you and your staff have identified at least six telephone calls related to transportation. One of your patients, Mr Koven, was hospitalized after an accident resulting from his making a faulty left turn. You had a call from the daughter of Mr Naka, who is concerned that her father, who has early-stage dementia, is no longer a safe driver; she wants you to talk to him about giving up his car keys. Mrs Rodriguez cancelled an appointment because her neighbor was unable to drive her to the appointment as planned. Mrs Lemke is a patient you have followed for many years, but she had to find a new physician because she moved into an assisted living facility that does not provide transportation to your clinic—it is beyond the geographic boundaries the facility serves. Although there are alternative transportation services available, there are some important limitations. Miss McKeg is one of your oldest patients. She uses a medical clinic transportation service, which is expensive. Furthermore, she has described her feelings of loss because she can no longer reliably get to activities that are important to her, including bridge games, volunteer work, and concerts. Mr Challes complained that it was very difficult to get the tests you prescribed because of inadequate parking at the lab. Although there was overflow parking, the distance was simply too far for him to walk, and all of the handicapped spaces were invariably taken. As you and your staff talk about these situations, you decide you will need to develop protocols and identify resources to address this increasingly important issue.

OPPORTUNITIES

Physicians are an important part of the interdisciplinary team that can address older adults' transportation issues. With respect to safety, drivers aged 85 or over are at the highest rate of crash risk per miles driven. Furthermore, mortality rates for these older drivers are extremely high.[1] Alternatives to driving may be limited in some communities, although a larger problem may be that older adults are unaware of services that exist or have no experience with public transportation and other transportation services and no knowledge of how to use them. Physicians, in partnership with other professionals, can assist older patients and their families navigate through changing transportation needs.

➤ Physicians can assess patients for conditions related to unsafe driving (eg, vision loss, recent acute events, chronic neurologic diseases, medications, and dementia), and provide appropriate information and counseling to patients and their family members about the impact of these conditions on driving.

➤ Physicians can provide exercises to older adults with chronic illnesses to help them maintain rapid reflexes, muscle strength, and flexibility.[2]

➤ Physicians can support family members and caregivers as they help unsafe drivers stop driving and find alternatives.

➤ Physicians play a key role in determining whether someone is unsafe to drive and, in some states, are required by law to report unsafe drivers. Physicians can assist as well with decisions about driving, including suggesting ways to improve safety and independence.

➤ Physicians can guide people to community resources that provide alternatives to driving and teach individuals or groups how to ride public transit.

➤ Physicians can participate in advocacy at their practices for adequate parking and signage, covered shelter while waiting for transport, and other supports for patients with disabilities.

➤ Physicians can help middle-aged and young-old patients think about and begin planning for future transportation needs.

➤ Physicians can work in partnership with other professionals to address patients' transportation needs. Examples include social workers to help identify community resources, to discuss feelings about making changes in transportation habits (eg, taking the bus instead of driving), or to resolve family conflicts around transportation issues; occupational therapists or kinesiotherapists for driver evaluation and rehabilitation; physical therapists for strength and balance training; audiologists for hearing assessment; ophthalmologists for vision testing; and advocates, planners, and legislators for needed public policy changes.

CHALLENGES

Giving up driving is extremely difficult for many older adults; it represents a loss of independence and an increase in dependency. Older adults with significant physical and cognitive impairment may be unaware of their unsafe driving practices. Furthermore, they may be resistant to conversations about their driving because of the implications for lost independence that accompany decisions or requirements to stop driving. Loss of driving negatively impacts emotional and psychological health. If alternative methods of transportation are not available, older adults can become isolated in their communities.

Older adults, compared to the younger population, make fewer trips and travel shorter distances. However, older adults complete 90% of their travel in private vehicles, with most traveling as drivers, not passengers.[3] Most older adults have been lifelong drivers with little or no experience with public transportation.

➤ Older adults are often unaware of public or private transportation options, other than driving, that are available.

➤ Even though older adults may worry about being stranded when they can no longer drive, they may not be willing to take public transportation.

➤ In communities with public transportation, schedules accommodate those in the workforce and may not be available in the middle of the day, on weekends, or at night.

➤ Older adults are more likely to walk to their destinations than those in other age groups, but there are negative safety implications given the lack of sidewalks or sidewalk connectivity in many communities. Poor maintenance can lead to hazards such as crowded, obstructed, or uneven sidewalks.[4,5]

➤ Access to public transportation may be limited for people with disabilities, in part because of the physical challenges of walking to and from transit stations or bus stops, waiting for buses without shelter or seating, boarding and alighting from buses, and transferring from one vehicle to another.

Alternatives to driving may be limited, depending on the community and the resources of the individual. Decisions about where to live are rarely made with future transportation needs in mind. In general, fewer alternatives are available in rural and suburban communities. Also, those living in less dense communities are less likely to leave their homes whether by walking or driving.[3]

➤ Older adults with medical conditions travel less, are more likely to ask for rides, and/or are more likely to limit driving to daylight hours.

➤ Assisted living and other types of senior housing are often built outside of urban centers, where public transportation is limited and zoning laws make it expensive to provide good transit services.

➤ Transportation services may be overburdened because demands often exceed available resources, resulting in unreliable services and frustrated patients, caregivers, and clinic staff.

Older adults with mobility problems may find any kind of transportation difficult, including trips to the physician, the grocery store, or recreational activities. Even with assistance from others, older adults with mobility problems may find it difficult to navigate from a car or bus up curbs and into a building without further assistance. In addition, those who rely on friends and families are often reluctant to become a burden; they may curtail or minimize trips, further isolating themselves or delaying needed services.

SOLUTIONS

Driver Safety

➤ Routinely assess older patients for conditions that impair driving; include screening for visual, musculoskeletal, and cognitive impairment and investigate the cause of such impairments and the potential for rehabilitation (a good example is the Assessment of Driving-Related Skills, a 10-minute office screening tool available at www.ama-assn.org/ama1/pub/upload/mm/433/phyguidechap3.pdf).[6]

➤ Ask older patients about their transportation needs and offer appropriate resource information (eg, keep brochures about local resources in the waiting area and in examination rooms).

➤ Consider working with patients to come to agreements about driving safety (eg, an advance directive for driving).[7] Include older adults in decision making; often when they are presented with objective information, they will make the decision to retire from driving.

➤ When appropriate, recommend to the Department of Motor Vehicles that limitations be placed on licenses of older adults with some impairment, such as limiting driving to daylight hours. Such limitations can reduce crash risk while allowing older drivers to maintain driving privileges.[8]

➤ Offer patients cognitive training targeting speed processing to help older adults maintain functional abilities, including driving. This has been effective in older adults who are at risk of mobility decline.[9]

➤ Refer patients to physical and occupational therapy to improve mobility.

➤ Suggest that patients enroll in driver refresher courses, such as that offered by AARP.[10]

➤ Refer patients to driver assessment and rehabilitation programs, which can provide driver education for older drivers to assist them to adapt safely to declining function. Sometimes vehicles can be fitted with adaptive equipment to facilitate driving (eg, foot brake extension, seating, hand controls).[11]

➤ Report any older adult who is an unsafe driver to the state licensing agency if mandated by state law and/or the patient is clearly an unsafe driver and is unlikely to stop driving on his/her own.

➤ Meet with family members to discuss your concerns (or theirs) about older family members who may be unsafe drivers. Resources such as *Driving Decisions in Later Life* can be very helpful for family members.[12]

Alternatives to Driving

If services that substitute for driving are convenient and easily accessible, older adults are more likely to use them. Provide information about resources and/or how to access transportation services (eg, alternatives to driving, older driver education, and rehabilitation services). To identify services in your community, check with your local Area Agency on Aging (to find the AAA, contact www.eldercare. gov, or call 800-677-1116). A variety of options exist in many communities:

➤ Public transportation such as buses may run on fixed, scheduled routes; some buses "kneel" to curb level or have low floors to make entry and exit easier.

➤ Flexible, on-demand transportation services specifically for older adults and/or people with disabilities are available in many areas; most of these programs, commonly known as "dial-a-ride" programs, provide curb-to-curb service, and some offer escort to and from the vehicle (door-to-door service) as well.

➤ Taxi services may specifically target people with disabilities.

➤ Volunteer driver programs exist in many communities. These senior/ volunteer escort or transportation services typically provide transport to medical appointments. Fewer provide transportation for recreational activities.

➤ Some older adults privately hire drivers (eg, the elder keeps the car and has friends or relatives drive it to transport him/her to activities, or the proceeds from the sale of the elder's car can go into a "travel account" that can be used to pay fares or drivers).

➤ Informal exchanges of services for transportation are arranged through families and friends.

➤ Motorized three-wheeled scooters or three-wheeled bicycles are feasible in some neighborhoods, particularly in communities designed for older adults.

Environmental Support

Physicians can make modifications to the physical environment of their practice to support older adults with mobility limitations.

➤ Ensure the clinic has an adequate number of designated handicapped parking spaces.

➤ Provide a sheltered entrance so that people who are dropped off are out of the weather as they exit the car.

➤ Provide a warm, dry place for patients to sit while they wait for their escorts to park the car and join them, or while they wait for transportation service drivers. Consider waiting areas that are accessible outside of clinic hours.

➤ Provide a wheelchair at the entrance.

➤ Ensure that automatic doors are installed and functioning.

Clinic Staff

Staff should be encouraged to anticipate and respond to patients' transportation and mobility needs:

➤ Ensure all staff are trained and available to address the needs of patients as they enter and leave the office/building (eg, assist with wheelchairs and doors).

➤ Ensure that staff who schedule appointments check the patient's chart for information on the person's ambulatory status (eg, needs standby assistance and/or uses cane, walker, or wheelchair) and ask about transportation arrangements at the time of making the appointment.

➤ Assist patients in calling for return rides if they are using a volunteer, taxi, or dial-a-ride service.

➤ Provide resource information about transportation options to older patients and their family members. Printed patient education materials in languages appropriate to your patient population may be provided in the waiting area.

➤ If patients rely on working family members or friends for transportation, consider the family member's needs when scheduling appointments (eg, at the beginning or end of the day).

➤ If patients rely on the assistance of a home health aide to get ready and get to the appointment, consider the aide's schedule and availability when scheduling the appointment.

➤ Balance the need to schedule multiple appointments (eg, to reduce number of trips made by family members) with patient fatigue.

➤ Maintain a petty cash fund for patients unable to pay cab fare as a backup option when other transportation arrangements fall through.

TAKE-HOME POINTS

➤ Transportation is a complex issue and is associated with quality of life.

➤ Normal age-related changes, as well as diseases and disabilities common in older adults, can adversely affect driving abilities.

➤ Physicians have a major role in assessing patients, providing information about options, working with professionals in other disciplines, and intervening when patients are no longer capable of driving safely.

USEFUL RESOURCES

AARP. *The Older Driver's Skill Assessment and Resource Guide: Creating Mobility Choices.* Publication No. D14957. AARP Fulfillment, PO Box 96796, Washington, DC 20090-6796.

American Automobile Association (AAA) Foundation for Traffic Safety. See www.seniordrivers.org for issues pertaining to seniors and their families; see http://AAASeniors.com for tips on "helping the senior driver in your life" make informed decisions on driving continuation or cessation.

American Medical Association in cooperation with the National Highway Traffic Safety Administration. *Physician's Guide to Assessing and Counseling Older Drivers.* 2010 (www.ama-assn.org/go/olderdrivers).

Ontario Ministry of Transportation. Senior Driver Group Education Curriculum (www.mto.gov.on.ca/english/dandv/driver/senior/senior.shtml).

REFERENCES

1. Odenheimer GL. Driver safety in older adults: the physician's role in assessing driving skills of older patients. *Geriatrics*. 2006;61(10):14–21.

2. American Society on Aging. Coordinating prevention and intervention: activities and services. Chapter 3. In: *Live Well, Live Long: Health Promotion and Disease Prevention for Older Adults – Road Map to Driving Wellness*. www.asaging.org/cdc/module4/phase3/index.cfm.

3. Neal M, Chapman N, Dill J, et al. Age-related shifts in housing and transportation demand: a multidisciplinary study conducted for Metro by Portland State University's College of Urban and Public Affairs. Portland, OR: Institute on Aging, Portland State University; August 14, 2006. www.pdx.edu/sites/www.pdx.edu.ioa/files/media_assets/cupa_age_related_shifts.pdf. Accessed February 4, 2010.

4. Rosenbloom S. Meeting transportation needs in an age-friendly community. *Generations*. 2009;33(2):33–43.

5. Neal MB, DeLaTorre A. The World Health Organization's Age-Friendly Cities Project in Portland, Oregon, USA (Summary of Findings). Portland, OR: Institute on Aging, Portland State University; October 1, 2007. www.pdx.edu/sites/www.pdx.edu.ioa/files/media_assets/ioa_age_friendly_cities.pdf.

6. AMA. Assessing functional abilities. Chapter 3. In: AMA Physician's Guide to Assessing and Counseling Older Drivers. www.ama-assn.org/ama/pub/physician-resources/public-health/promoting-healthy-lifestyles/geriatric-health/older-driver-safety/assessing-counseling-older-drivers.shtml. Accessed February 4, 2010.

7. Odenheimer GL. Driver safety in older adults: the physician's role in assessing driving skills of older patients. *Geriatrics*. 2006;61(10):14–21.

8. Nasvadi GC, Wister A. Do restricted driver's licenses lower crash risk among older drivers? A survival analysis of insurance data from British Columbia. *Gerontologist*. 2009;49:474–484.

9. Edwards JD, Myers C, Ross LA, et al. The longitudinal impact of cognitive speed of processing training on driving mobility. *Gerontologist*. 2009;49:485–494.

10. AARP Online Driver Safety Program [free online course]. www.aarpdriversafety.org. Accessed February 4, 2010.

11. Staplin L, Hunt L. Driver programs. In: Conference Proceedings, November 7–9, 1999: Transportation in an Aging Society: A Decade of Experience. Washington, DC: Transportation Research Board of the National Academies; 2004. http://onlinepubs.trb.org/onlinepubs/conf/reports/cp_27.pdf#page=82. Accessed February 4, 2010.

12. Schmall VL, Bowman S, Vorhies DG. *Driving Decisions in Later Life*. 1998. http://openlibrary.org/b/OL16048586M/Driving_decisions_in_later_life. Accessed February 4, 2010.

CHAPTER EIGHTEEN

Medication Refills

Kristy Butler, PharmD, BCPS

Ian Ferrari, PharmD candidate

MRS BLEWITT'S EXPERIENCE

Mrs Blewitt has settled into her new assisted living environment and seems to be making slow but steady improvement in her cognitive function and mobility. You have started her on Donepezil and this seems to have improved her ability to perform her own activities of daily living. Now that Mrs Blewitt has medication management (providing administration supervision and communications regarding refills or side effects) at her facility, you have changed all her medications to 3-month supplies with a mail-order pharmacy. At your last visit, you added Memantine, but her son called back a few days later to report a problem. The assisted living facility charges $18 each time they provide dosing assistance to patients, so Mrs Blewitt's medication charge has gone from $540 per month to $1080 per month—just to supervise administering her drugs. You decide together with the patient and son to forgo the trial of Memantine for now, and Mrs Blewitt continues to do well thanks to her engaged clinic team, care facility, and loving family.

OPPORTUNITIES

Helping people make the best use of medications is a core mission of clinical pharmacists. The recommendations presented in this chapter come from the perspective of pharmacists who have practiced in a variety of health care settings, including ambulatory clinics, community pharmacies, and acute care hospitals.

Older adults are the biggest consumers of medications, with more than 93% of adults older than 65 years using at least one medication (prescription or nonprescription drug, vitamin/mineral, herbal/natural supplement), 57% to 59% using more than five, and 17% to 19% taking at least 10 in a given week.[1] Although the prevalence of overall medication use has remained stable among older adults, the rate of polypharmacy (ie, the use of 5 or more medications) has increased compared to a decade ago.[2] In addition to increased use of medications, changes in medication metabolism and sensitivity to medication side effects place older adults at increased risk for medication adverse effects and drug-drug interactions. This highly variable and vulnerable population can also experience sudden changes to their health status, and medication changes (dose adjustments, discontinuation of medications, adding other medications) can occur frequently. Given all of these factors, a thorough review and reconciliation of all prescription and nonprescription medications should be completed at each patient encounter, including telephone refill/medication requests, office visits, and hospitalizations.

Nearly 50% of all non–office-based encounters in ambulatory practices involve refill requests.[3] When optimized (see Solutions below), the medication refill process can provide the following benefits for practices caring for older adults:

➤ *Improved patient adherence.* Ensuring patients have timely access to their medications (particularly long-standing medications for stable chronic conditions) can improve medication adherence.[4–6]

➤ *Improved patient safety.* Standardized protocols may decrease medication errors by including an evaluation of safety and monitoring parameters (laboratory tests, drug-drug interactions, contraindications, inappropriate dosing, etc). They may also decrease gaps in treatment.[6]

➤ *Improved effectiveness.* Reviewing goals of therapy can be included in the refill process, identifying opportunities to optimize therapy.[7]

➤ *Improved efficiency.* Standardized protocols have demonstrated faster turnaround times, decreased repeat refill requests, and decreased prescriber time and effort on refill approvals, allowing more time for direct patient care.[8] Separate protocols may be considered for unique populations (geriatrics vs adults vs pediatrics, specialty clinics vs general medicine, etc). Standardization should only be used to the extent that it benefits the patient; teams need to apply critical thinking to anticipate and prevent harm.

➤ *Improved patient satisfaction.* Patients express satisfaction with faster approval of refills and fewer repeat requests.[4]

➤ *Improved staff satisfaction.* In some refill processes, support staff team members are given more responsibility, allowing them to practice at the top of their license/scope of practice as permitted by law and practice policy.

➤ *Improved prescriber satisfaction.* A standardized process can decrease prescribers' paperwork, allow more time to focus on direct patient care, and possibly reduce after-hours "urgent" refill requests.[9]

CHALLENGES

Despite these advantages, there are challenges associated with the medication refill process, particularly in older patients:

➤ Refill requests often take a significant amount of time and resources.[6,8]

➤ Refill requests often occur outside of patient visits and, under current fee-for-service reimbursement models, are not compensated, despite clinical assessment and decision making that may take place.[3]

➤ Without standardized systems in place, there is often wide variability in workflow and practices around the refill process. This can lead to delays, medication errors, lack of monitoring, and other quality issues.[6,8]

➤ Use of refill protocols (see Solutions below) requires a willingness to change workflows, increase staff responsibility, give up provider control, and devote time to planning, training, implementation, and evaluation.

➤ Increased responsibilities and tasks for clinical support staff may be met with resistance or may require other tasks to be reprioritized or reassigned.

➤ There may be an initial decline in efficiency when a new workflow and protocols are first implemented. Some staff may require additional training or oversight during implementation.

➤ Legal requirements based on state and federal regulations must be followed in any protocol.

SOLUTIONS

Access to Medications

Ensure patients have timely access to their medications (particularly medications for chronic conditions).

➤ Barriers to timely access could include transportation to and from the pharmacy, refills not being ready (suggest the patient call the pharmacy to ensure the prescription is ready before going to pick it up), prescription cost/ insurance coverage issues (suggest optimizing use of generic and preferred brand medications when possible, or consider offering samples or coupons if available to cover period of waiting for nonpreferred medications).

➤ Consider prescribing a 3-month supply of medications and longer refills (1- or 2-year refills) for long-term medications.[10] Long-term medications might include treatments for chronic conditions such as thyroid supplementation, diabetes medications and supplies, antihypertensive and lipid-lowering therapies, inhalers for chronic obstructive pulmonary disease or asthma, and bisphosphonates. Periodic review of long-term medications for appropriate dose and ongoing use is always recommended.

➤ Consider use of mail-order pharmacies or automatic refill services at the pharmacy (depending on patient preference and/or insurance requirements) to prevent gaps in medication use.[10]

➤ Review all medications and consider approving refills of all long-term medications rather than only the few that the patient or pharmacy may be requesting that day.

➤ Attempt to work with the patient's pharmacy to get medications filled on the same schedule. This can be challenging from an insurance perspective—the patient may need to pay for a small prescription of a few medications to get all their medications to run out at the same time—but is worth the effort. Consider offering samples or coupons to help bridge the interval to next refill and facilitate synchronizing multiple refills (if available).

Refill Protocols

Standardized refill protocols are increasingly being used to facilitate the authorization of refills for certain medications by nonprescribers (eg, clinical support staff).[5,8,9,11] The following are steps that can be taken to achieve an expedient, efficient, and safe process that will enhance patient, staff, and provider satisfaction; improve cost-effectiveness; and improve patient adherence to medication regimens. All protocols should be considered within the context of your state regulatory requirements for practitioners licensed to manage prescriptions.

1. Under the supervision of a licensed independent practitioner, clinical support staff may approve prescription refill requests (of certain medication classes) provided that both patient-specific and prescription-specific criteria have been met.

2. Develop a refill protocol (software programs are also available for purchase).

   a. Included (and excluded) medications/classes

      i. Include required laboratory tests and time frames.

      ii. Note special issues (how many refills can be authorized—1 year from last appointment or laboratory tests, 3 months, etc).

      iii. In a geriatric practice, appropriate classes of medications—and how many refills may be authorized—may differ from those in an adult medicine practice.

   b. Patient-specific requirements

      i. Patient is established or "active" in practice. Definitions vary, but many practices require at least one office encounter (and no notification of transfer of care to another provider) in past 2 to 3 years to maintain "active" status with the clinic.

      ii. Last office visit is within a designated period (ie, previous 12 months).

   c. Prescription-specific requirements

      i. Requested refill is for a medication active and current on medication list (including exact medication, dose, and directions).

      ii. Date of refill request is appropriate (within acceptable time frame, not excessively early or late).

      iii. There is no documentation in patient's chart of allergy, adverse drug reaction, drug-drug interaction, or contraindication to the medication.

      iv. Required laboratory testing has been completed within time frame indicated in protocol, and results of those tests are within normal limits.

   d. Provider, clinic, and institution approval

3. Workflow development

   a. Include tools to facilitate standardized process and improve efficiency (ie, forms, templates, text).

   b. Refill requests that fall outside of the clinical and safety parameters are forwarded to the prescriber (or in some cases, doctor of pharmacy) for review and action. If the patient is overdue for laboratory tests or an appointment, support staff may contact the patient to schedule and approve a 1-month supply of some medications, according to protocol.

   c. Appropriate documentation is performed.[12]

   d. Prescriber cosigns all approved refills.

4. Implementation/spread

   a. Plan for training time for staff.

   b. Ensure that support staff team members are available to do the refills; the protocol will not work if team members are already overworked.

   c. Consider small pilots with limited staff and medication classes.

Quality assurance must be built into the implementation (all refills done by newly trained staff should be reviewed until accuracy is ensured).[13,14]

Other Tips and Tricks

➤ Simplify dosing regimen (once-daily dosing, combine drugs into one tablet when possible and if cost allows).[15]

➤ Encourage use of prefilled pill boxes, bubble packs, or "salad packs" to help patients stay organized and improve self-management skills and adherence.[10]

➤ Good communication is paramount.[7,16] When a patient starts a new medication, he or she should have the following questions answered:

  ➤ What are the goals of therapy? Stress the importance of medication in disease management and when the medication should start to take effect.

  ➤ What are the expected (common) side effects, and rare or serious adverse drug events? Give special attention to effects that may change the patient's stability, cognition, bathroom use frequency, appetite, sleep, or mood.

  ➤ What is the expected duration of therapy?

  ➤ When is follow-up needed for side effects and therapeutic outcomes? This includes telephone management, office visits, or laboratory tests that are needed for monitoring.

  ➤ What is the expected cost of the medication? There are many resources (pharmacy and drug store Web sites, online formularies, online services for physicians such as Epocrates (www.epocrates.com) that can provide this information.

➤ If the patient lives in a facility, print out an extra copy of the new medication list and orders after the visit for the patient to give to the facility.

➤ If the patient uses mail order, be sure to get the name of a local pharmacy for urgent medications or refills needed before the mail-order supply can be received.

➤ Ask patients to request refills from their pharmacy rather than calling your office.[12] Patients should, however, be encouraged to contact your office any time they have questions, problems, life changes, or other information that may affect medication safety or use.

➤ Request that pharmacies fax or use e-prescribing to request refills from the clinic.[12]

➤ Clinic staff should call the patient if a refill is denied (or a laboratory test or appointment is due).[12] The pharmacy should call the patient when the refill is ready.

➤ Advise the use of a single pharmacy. Using a single pharmacy makes it easier for the physician and the pharmacy alike to track progress as well as drug-drug and drug-disease interactions and potentially reduces confusion for everyone. If a patient needs to use a separate pharmacy for some items such as compounded medications, infusions, or "specialty" medications, encourage the patient to provide all pharmacies and prescribers a complete medication list. Future advances in electronic prescribing may assist medication reconciliation across different prescribers and pharmacies as well.

➤ Verify that patients have appropriate health literacy to read medication labels and take their medications as prescribed; use the "teach back" method to determine whether the patient can demonstrate understanding and use the information conveyed. Ask patients to bring all medications in the prescription vials to visits to verify how they are taking the medication and whether they know how to read the label to identify pertinent information (eg, quantity, refills remaining, instructions, and expiration date).[16] Consider having patients demonstrate how they go about identifying their medication.

➤ Utilize community-, clinic-, or hospital-based pharmacy services for medication reconciliation and management as a component of best practice.[5,9–11,17,18]

TAKE-HOME POINTS

➤ Medication refills take time and resources, but they can be an opportunity to improve patient self-management, adherence, medication safety, and team-based care.

➤ A standardized refill process in the office has the potential to improve many aspects of care, especially in practices caring for older adults.

REFERENCES

1. Patterns of medication use in the United States, 2006: a report from the Slone Survey. www.bu.edu/slone/SloneSurvey/AnnualRpt/SloneSurveyWebReport2006.pdf. Accessed February 5, 2010.

2. Gurwitz JH, Field TS, Harrold LR, et al. Incidence and preventability of adverse drug events among older persons in the ambulatory setting. *JAMA*. 2003;289(9):1107–1116.

3. Spencer DC, Daugird AJ. The nature and content of telephone prescribing habits in a community practice. *Fam Med*. 1990;22:205–209.

4. Shapiro NL, Breen M, Mategrano VA. Patient satisfaction with a scheduled prescription-refill service. *Am J Health Syst Pharm.* 2001;58(4):322–325.

5. VA telephone care program gives pharmacists authority to solve zero-refill problem. *Clin Resour Manag.* 2000;1(8):120–123, 113.

6. Escobedo J. Rethinking refills. *Fam Pract Manage.* 2002;9(9):55.

7. Kennedy J, Tuleu I, Mackay K. Unfilled prescriptions of Medicare beneficiaries: prevalence, reasons, and types of medicines prescribed. *J Manag Care Pharm.* 2008;14(6):553–560.

8. Gerdes M. Chronic disease tracking using a refill protocol. November 11, 2009. http://blogs.aafp.org/fpm/transformation/entry/chronic_disease_tracking_using_a.

9. Cassidy IB, Keith MR, Coffey EL, et al. Impact of pharmacist-operated general medicine chronic care refill clinics on practitioner time and quality of care. *Ann Pharmacother.* 1996;30:745–750.

10. Gross R, Zhang Y, Grossberg R. Medication refill logistics and refill adherence in HIV. *Pharmacoepidemiol Drug Saf.* 2005;14(11):789–793.

11. Jones RJ, Goldman MP, Rockwood RP, et al. Beneficial effect of a pharmacy refill evaluation clinic. *Hosp Pharm.* 1987;22:166–168.

12. Ferrell CW, Aspy CB, Mold JW. Management of prescription refills in primary care: an Oklahoma Physicians Resource/Research Network (OKPRN) study. *J Am Board Fam Med.* 2006;19(1):31–38.

13. Cram DL, Maesner AT, Witmore DM. Medication refill clinics: the Veterans Administration Medical Center experience. *J Pharm Pract.* 1992;5(1):12–21.

14. Cram DL, Stebbins M, Eom S, et al. Peer review as a quality assurance mechanism in three pharmacist-run medication-refill clinics. *Am J Hosp Pharm.* 1992;49:2727–2730.

15. Munger MA, Van Tassell BW, LaFleur J. Medication nonadherence: an unrecognized cardiovascular risk factor. *Med Gen Med.* 2007;9(3):58.

16. Akici A, Kalaca S, Ugurlu MU, Toklu HZ, Iskender E, Oktay S. Patient knowledge about drugs prescribed at primary healthcare facilities. *Pharmacoepidemiol Drug Saf.* 2004;13(12):871–876.

17. Helling DK, Nelson KM, Ramirez JE, Humphries TL. Kaiser Permanente Colorado Region Pharmacy Department: innovative leader in pharmacy practice. *J Am Pharm Assoc.* 2006;46(1):67–76.

18. Riege VJ. A patient safety program & research evaluation of U.S. Navy pharmacy refill clinics. In: Henriksen K, Battles JB, Marks ES, Lewin DI, eds. *Advances in Patient Safety, Vol 1: Research Findings.* AHRQ publication No. 05-0021-1. Rockville, MD: Agency for Healthcare Research and Quality; February 2005.

CHAPTER NINETEEN

Tips for Small Practices: Lessons Learned From Care Management Implementation

Melinda Davis, MA, PhD candidate

Monica Goubaud, MA, CCRP

Lyle J. (L.J.) Fagnan, MD

CLINICIAN EXPERIENCE

You are the co-owner of a small physician-owned primary care clinic. During the last 10 years your practice has often been the sole source of primary care in the local community. As in many areas, the demographics of your community and your practice mirror the nation's aging population. Additionally, it seems that access to community-based support services is dwindling. Personally, you are feeling the challenges of trying to manage older, more complex patients with multiple chronic conditions during 15-minute appointments. Your patients frequently present with mental health concerns (although they are too proud to call it depression). One patient in particular, whom you recently diagnosed with mild cognitive impairment, has required numerous efforts to coordinate her care.

In your continuing medical education activities you've read about the patient-centered medical home and suggestions for utilizing team-based care. Since patients older than 65 make up more than 23% of your patient panel, you've started thinking about the potential for integrating care management and care coordination in your practice as a way to help manage your senior patients, as well as other high-risk populations. You've seen evidence that care coordination and nurse-based care management had positive clinical and economic outcomes in a large health system[1] and its associated primary care clinics.[2] However, you are having trouble finding research exploring the economic and social implications of integrating care management in smaller primary care settings, even though three-fourths of primary care practices employ five or fewer physicians.[3] Given this context, you wonder how your clinic could afford to create this new position, how you'd find someone qualified for this role that you could trust, and what it would take to incorporate care management into your practice.

Early in your career you practiced with a clinician who is now on faculty at the state university and directs a practice-based research network. Given that practice-based research networks engage practicing primary care clinicians in collaborative research about issues relevant to routine care delivery,[4] you think he might be a good source of advice. When you reach him he reports that he recently completed a project to incorporate Care Management Plus (CMP) into six small, rural primary care practices.[5] He offered to share with you the following lessons learned through feedback from interviews conducted with four practice cohorts (clinician champions, clinicians, administrators, and nurse care managers) before the CMP intervention and approximately 1 year after the intervention, along with the observations of the research team.

OPPORTUNITIES

The concept of care management, as a component of the patient-centered medical home, presents an ideal opportunity to enhance long-term care delivery in a primary care system that is organized to address acute medical concerns. The CMP model utilizes information technology and facilitates team-based care through the use of a nurse care manager. Nurse care managers work to address the needs and preference of older adults and those with complex medical conditions by assisting with chronic disease management, providing patient education, and coordinating care.

Clinics engaged in the CMP study with the goals that integrating or enhancing nurse care managers in their practices would include both intermediate (eg, improved communication) and bottom line (eg, cost savings) outcomes, such as the following:

➤ Better care coordination and patient follow-up

➤ Improved quality of care (demonstrated by patient outcomes)

➤ Increased clinic efficiency

➤ Improved team care

➤ Increased patient self-management

➤ Enhanced communication through health information technology

Clinics that implemented CMP reported many of these items as successful outcomes, including incorporating care management into routine care, receiving positive responses from clinician and patient users of nurse care managers, developing a systematic way to track care and communicate outcomes, improved patient care, and enhanced links to clinical/community services.

CHALLENGES

There are many characteristics of smaller clinical practices that make it both easier and more frightening to explore the possibility of change. Challenges to implementing CMP included addressing both the typical barriers to treating chronic diseases in primary care (ie, provider and staffing limitations, inadequate systems for population management, and the general payment structure) as well as the complexities of managing substantial practice change. As one family physician said in exasperation about delivering chronic care services, "I'm just trying to keep them alive this week."

In addition to system barriers, various challenges stemmed directly from the changes associated with implementing CMP. These include redefining team roles and getting clinic-wide buy-in, balancing limited clinic resources (finances, time, staffing), and learning new information technology systems (or how to use present systems). Change itself was identified as a barrier; all four practice cohorts commented that change can be tiring, that it is "generally resisted," and that having the "time to change" can be a problem. As one clinician noted, resistance to change tends to be the case *even if* things are not currently being done well.

STRATEGIES AND RECOMMENDATIONS FOR SUCCESS

Despite the challenges associated with implementing CMP, the clinics had thoughtful advice to facilitate success. With the caveat that all health care delivery is local and your clinic will have unique features that will need consideration when implementing CMP or other practice changes, the following tips may be helpful:

1. Get administrative buy-in.

    ➤ If you're the practice owner, this is easy—it's your call.

    ➤ If you are a co-owner or part of a hospital-owned system, be sure that those who control decision making and resource allocation get on board with this project. Having the support of administration is an essential piece to getting CMP off the ground and flourishing.

2. Network—you don't have to do this work alone.

    ➤ Connect with peers who have worked or are currently working to improve care coordination or implement care management. Locate these clinics by attending regional meetings or by picking up the telephone. Don't re-create the wheel if you don't have to.

    ➤ Explore opportunities for affiliation with a practice-based research network out of a nearby university or with other health improvement agencies. These groups might have "practice facilitators" who serve as external agents to encourage or guide change.[6]

3. Find the right person for the job of care manager (CM)—and clarify roles across the practice.

    ➤ Many of the sites attributed the successful implementation of care management to "having the right person for the job."

    ➤ Look at your current staff. Is there someone who could assume these responsibilities if he or she received brief training in care management?

    ➤ Look for someone who is organized, a good communicator, and willing to learn new skills. The CMP practices found that RNs were well suited for the job, but the right LPN, social worker, diabetes educator, or experienced medical assistant can also be a good fit.

    ➤ Adding the new position will require redefining or clarifying roles within the practice, both for the CM and for others who may have done some of these tasks in the past.

    ➤ This is an outstanding opportunity to facilitate clinician, nursing staff, and others to practice at the top of their license. For example, the CM can provide patient education that was previously done by the clinician, and medical assistants can be taught to "scrub charts" to identify needed clinical preventive services or to conduct the Personal Health Questionnaire two-question depression screen when placing a patient in a room.

➤ It is vital that you budget time for the CM to perform his or her new role. If you "hire" a current employee to serve as the CM, be sure to delegate some of that employee's current tasks to others. If the CM does not have any time to coordinate care, he or she will not coordinate care.

4. Market the new position.

➤ *To the clinic:* Provide leadership and describe the vision of the new model for chronic illness care in your practice. Share the CM job description around the practice and clarify how this role differs from that of the staff nurse or medical assistant. Consider hosting an open house where staff and clinicians can mingle with the CM, ask questions, and learn about the referral process.

➤ *To the patients:* Studies show that patients are appreciative of the efforts of the CM. They appreciate the opportunity to connect with a member in the clinic and to have someone assist in addressing their social and medical needs. We found that introductions work best with a "warm handoff" (ie, when the provider walks a patient down the hall or calls the CM in for a personal introduction).

➤ *To the community:* Provide the CM with time to identify and network with local agencies. This is an ideal opportunity for the CM to learn about existing resources while clarifying his or her role and responsibilities for community partners. In small communities, be sure to have a time frame for the position; a longer commitment will encourage community members to take the time to invest in the relationship.

5. Target patient populations with implementation.

➤ You may want your care manager to partner in the management of all your patients. However, we recommend starting small by selecting a subset of your patient population for the CM to work with initially. This may be based on a diagnosis that the CM has experience working with (eg, the CM is a diabetes educator) or one that makes up the majority of your panel.

➤ Select two or three quality measures that you can track. This will help you gather hard data that you can use to market the CM services to other members of the clinic.

➤ Not all patients respond well to care management. If things aren't working, don't push it. Let patients know that the CM's door is open should they be interested in the future.

6. Be patient.

> ➤ Practice change takes time, and it is an iterative process. Besides the day-to-day time requirements, research indicates that practice change takes longer than 12 to 24 months.[7-9]

> ➤ Take it slow so you are able to learn from your failures, and remember to celebrate your successes.

USEFUL RESOURCES

Mohler PJ, Mohler NB. Improving chronic illness care: lessons learned in a private practice. *Fam Pract Manage.* 2005;50–56.

Johns Hopkins University. Practice leaders in medical homes (www.medhomeinfo.org/tools/physiciancourse/index.html).

REFERENCES

1. Dorr DA, Wilcox AB, Brunker CP, et al. The effect of technology-supported, multidisease care management on the mortality and hospitalization of seniors. *JAGS.* 2008;56(12):2195–2202.

2. Dorr DA, Wilcox A, McConnell J, et al. Productivity enhancement for primary care providers using multicondition care management. *Am J Managed Care.* 2007;13(1):20–27.

3. Hing E, Burt CW. Characteristics of office-based physicians and their practices: United States, 2005–2006. *Vital Health Stat.* 2008;13(166):1–34.

4. Mold JW, Pasternak A, McCaulay A, et al. Definitions of common terms relevant to primary care research. *Ann Fam Med.* 2008;6:570–571.

5. Care Management Plus: Information Technology Tools for the Care of Seniors. http://caremanagementplus.org. Accessed November 14, 2009.

6. Nagykaldi Z, Mold JW, Robinson A, et al. Practice facilitators and practice-based research networks. *J Am Board Fam Med.* 2006;19(5):506–510.

7. Counsell SR, Callahan CM, Clark DO, et al. Geriatric care management for low-income seniors: a randomized controlled trial. *JAMA.* 2007;298(22):2623–2633.

8. Gagnon AJ, Schein C, McVey L, Bergman H. Randomized controlled trial of nurse case management of frail older people. *J Am Geriatr Soc.* 1999;47(9):1118–1124.

9. Sledge WH, Brown KE, Levine JM, et al. A randomized trial of primary intensive care to reduce hospital admissions in patients with high utilization of inpatient services. *Dis Manag.* 2006;9(6):328–338.

CHAPTER | TWENTY

Organizing a Community of Geriatric Primary Care Providers

David Mehr, MD, MS

PHYSICIAN EXPERIENCE

A physician, who is medical director of a primary care clinic and serves as the physician consultant to a nearby assisted living facility, observes that 13 patients died during a recent influenza outbreak in the community and the facility. He contacts several other medical directors and providers active in the area. After reviewing Centers for Disease Control and Prevention guidelines, they agree on a protocol for instituting prophylactic antiviral therapy if there is an influenza outbreak in their associated facilities. They circulate this suggested protocol to their colleagues who care for nursing home, assisted living, and other community residents. When the next influenza outbreak is recognized, each facility contacts providers to ask whether the protocol should be implemented for their patients.

INTRODUCTION

There are multiple strategies toward improving care of older adults with complex medical needs. The main focus of this chapter is to discuss bringing together providers of care for older adults within a community. However, for particularly vulnerable older adults, such as those with multiple chronic conditions, several geriatric care models have been developed, which may be available in some locales.

Most of these programs include care coordination or management, often by a nurse or nurse practitioner. This care coordinator is usually supported by a geriatric team that works with the primary physician. Some of these geriatric models of care, such as the Geriatric Resources for Assessment and Care of Elders (GRACE) program, IMPACT for depression management, or Care Management Plus (See Useful Resources section at the end of this chapter for references) have shown cost savings in addition to improved quality of care. Another care model focuses on care transitions across settings of care. Again frequently involving a nurse, care transition programs attempt to ensure that there is a seamless transition of care across settings, such as hospital to home. Programs may involve home visits or, at a minimum, telephone follow-up to identify problems, which are particularly likely to occur with medications. With new Medicare rules potentially penalizing hospitals for early readmissions, hospitals may find it financially worthwhile to support care transition programs. The Care Transitions Project provides a wealth of information on this important area of care. See Table 20-1 for a summary of additional models of care that have shown lower costs, use of health service, or improved quality for care for older adults.

OPPORTUNITIES

Bringing community geriatric providers together can provide a useful resource for tackling a specific problem or future issues. Beyond a common influenza protocol, a community of providers caring for nursing home patients, for example, could also collaborate on establishing uniform policies on resuscitation, information needed for transfers, and research projects. However, collaboration is certainly not restricted to the nursing home setting. Providers can organize to meet on a regular basis to discuss common issues or promote continuing education. This collaboration could arise independently with interest from a few individuals or could be combined with periodic meetings of a state chapter of the American Geriatrics Society or the American Medical Directors Association. They could unite to participate in a community-wide initiative to improve care for a geriatric syndrome or a specific chronic disease. For example, working in conjunction with the Alzheimer's Association or using established guidelines, providers could identify useful tools for providing quality dementia care and for identifying local community resources that would be useful to caregivers. Disease-specific organizations, such as the Alzheimer's Association, are often eager to share information and resources.

The developing interest in medical home models and planned demonstrations may provide another avenue for geriatric primary care providers to share expertise.

TABLE 20-1 Ambulatory models of care for older adults

	Potential benefits
Specific care management	Lower use/costs of health services; improved quality of care/life, survival, and functional autonomy
Interdisciplinary primary care	Lower use of health services; improved quality of care/life, functional autonomy, and survival
Pharmaceutical care	Lower use of health services; improved quality of care/life and survival
Chronic disease self-management training	Lower use/costs of health services; improved quality of life and functional autonomy
Proactive rehabilitation	Improved quality of life, functional autonomy, and survival
Caregiver education and support	Lower use/costs of health services; improved quality of life and functional autonomy
Transitional care	Lower use/costs of health services; improved quality of life and survival
Disease management	Lower use of health services; improved quality of care/life, functional autonomy, and survival
Preventive home visits	Lower use/costs of health services; improved functional autonomy and survival

Adapted from Boult C, Green AF, et al. Successful models of comprehensive care for older adults with chronic conditions: evidence for the Institute of Medicine's 'Retooling for an Aging America' report. *JAGS*. 2009;57:2328–2337.

Current procedures for gaining certification as a medical home can be complex and time consuming (see Chapter 23 for basics on the medical home). However, demonstration programs and possible more widespread initiatives in the future may require it. Providers can share experience and resources in gaining certification or collaborate to work on the process together with support from the American Geriatrics Society or primary care organizations. Theoretically, and in a few instances in practice, providers could also work together to share resources to support a medical home model.

CHALLENGES

Although most providers are motivated to see improvements in care, often the realities of a busy practice militate against taking on additional activities. Moreover, agreement may not be as simple as agreeing to adopt a national guideline.

Medical home demonstration projects are highly variable and may involve one payer or multiple. Whether or not collaborating around participation is feasible will be highly dependent on place and time. The most fundamental barrier is that participating with other providers is outside of usual work flows and does not contribute to financial reimbursement.

SOLUTIONS

Most physicians can get together over a meal at least occasionally to discuss an important topic. Use of good meeting principles, such as having an advance agenda and setting time limits on specific items, can greatly facilitate effective use of time. There is no substitute for an effective and motivated leader. If possible, having a working document or convening a very small and motivated group to create a working document is facilitative.

In the short term, focused projects that work on a well-defined limited issue, such as responding to an influenza outbreak, are most feasible. Regularly connecting providers to discuss important issues linked to continuing education is also something that occurs in selected communities now.

As the health care environment changes, more opportunities may develop to formally organize groups of providers and share scarce resources, such as working together on medical home certification or case management assistance. Such undertakings require careful organization.

USEFUL RESOURCES

American Geriatrics Society (AGS) (www.americangeriatrics.org).

American Medical Directors Association (AMDA) (www.amda.com/).

Alzheimer's Association (www.alz.org).

Geriatric care models:

➤ Care Management Plus (http://caremanagementplus.org/).

➤ GRACE Program (www.medicine.iupui.edu/IUCAR/research/grace.asp).

➤ IMPACT depression management (http://impact-uw.org/).

➤ Care Transitions Project (www.caretransitions.org/).

CHAPTER | TWENTY-ONE

Guided Care

Chad Boult, MD, MPH, MBA
Tracy Novak, MHS

MR JOHNSON'S EXPERIENCE

Ben Johnson is an 82-year-old, widowed, retired teacher who has been living on Social Security, a modest pension, and traditional fee-for-service Medicare. He has hypertension, diabetes, heart failure, mild cognitive impairment, osteoarthritis, and depression, for which he takes eight prescription medications each day. His daughter, Marie, who lives across town with three teenage children and works as an elementary school teacher, is Mr Johnson's primary source of assistance and emotional support.

Mr Johnson sees Dr Lynn Lewis, his primary care physician, every 3 months and a cardiologist and an orthopedist two to three times per year. Unfortunately, exacerbations of heart failure have required Mr Johnson to be hospitalized three times during the past year, each followed by 2 weeks at a skilled nursing facility and several weeks of home health care. Each time he has returned home, Mr Johnson has been weak, depressed, and confused about the medications he should take and the diet he should follow. Stressed by the many tasks involved in caring for her father and her children, Marie has decreased her teaching (and her income) by 50% and is considering placing her father in a nursing home.

Dr Lewis is concerned that Mr Johnson may not be safe living alone and that he may not be taking all of his prescribed medications correctly and adhering to his low-salt diet. She is also not sure what medications, diet, and activities Mr Johnson's other doctors have prescribed. Dr Lewis wishes there were more time to talk with Mr Johnson and his daughter, but the office visits last barely long enough to do a cursory physical examination and renew the necessary prescriptions.

OPPORTUNITIES

Guided Care is a care coordination model that was designed to improve the quality of care and the quality of life for people like Mr Johnson. It also aims to reduce the burden for caregivers like Marie, to improve the professional satisfaction of physicians like Dr Lewis, and to reduce total health care costs. In creating the Guided Care model, a multidisciplinary clinical team at The Johns Hopkins University infused into primary care the most current evidence-based guidelines for managing chronic conditions and the most effective principles from case management, disease management, self-management, transitional care, geriatric evaluation, and caregiver support models.

Guided Care is a model of proactive, comprehensive health care for people with several chronic conditions. In Guided Care, a specially trained registered nurse, based in a primary care practice, works closely with three to four physicians to provide state-of-the-art care for 50 to 60 chronically ill patients. These patients are members of the practice's panel whose risk of heavy health care use during the next year is in the top 20% to 25% (computed from insurance claims using the Hierarchical Condition Category predictive model). After a comprehensive home assessment and an evidence-based care planning process (described in detail by Boyd[1]), the Guided Care nurse monitors patients monthly, promotes self-management, smoothes transitions between sites of care, educates and supports family caregivers, facilitates access to community resources, and coordinates the efforts of health care professionals, hospitals, and community agencies to avoid duplication and to ensure that no important health-related issue slips through the cracks.

Current research has shown that Guided Care improves the quality of chronic care and physicians' satisfaction with chronic care processes, and it reduces caregivers' strain and insurers' expenditures for health care.

CHALLENGES

Although Guided Care improves chronic care, practices interested in adopting this model need to determine whether they can meet five requirements.

1. *Panel size:* The patient population needs to be large enough to contain 50 to 60 patients with several chronic conditions. Panels of at least 300 Medicare patients are usually sufficient. Practices with larger panels may be able to support more than one Guided Care nurse. Practices with smaller panels could share a Guided Care nurse if they were in proximity to each other.

2. *Office space:* A small, private, centrally located office is needed for the nurse. An ideal location is near the physicians' offices with convenient access to the practice's staff, medical records, supplies, and office equipment.

3. *Health information technology:* A locally installed or Web-based health information technology system is required.

4. *Commitment:* The practice's physician(s) and office staff members need to work collaboratively with the Guided Care nurse. Integration of a new type of health care provider into a primary care practice is a process that requires careful planning, optimism, open communication, honest feedback, flexibility, perseverance, and patience.

5. *Supplemental revenue:* Guided Care generates significant costs for the practice: the nurse's salary and benefits, office space, equipment (eg, computer, cell phone), communication services (eg, cell phone service, access to the Internet), and travel costs. To adopt Guided Care, a practice must be confident that it will receive a supplemental revenue stream that will offset these costs; for example, the Centers for Medicare and Medicaid Services' capitated care management payments to practices that participate in the proposed Medicare Medical Home Demonstration would more than cover the practice's costs related to employing a Guided Care nurse.

SOLUTIONS

Guided Care is a well-defined model of care that primary care practices can fully implement in 6 to 9 months. There are five critical steps in implementing Guided Care.

1. Preparing the Physicians and Office Staff

It is important to introduce and explain Guided Care clearly to the physicians and practice staff and describe how it will work in the practice. Staff members should understand how they will need to adjust some established roles and procedures to collaborate effectively with the Guided Care nurse. Some of the information that should be communicated is outlined below.

1. Guided Care introduction

   a. Inform attendees that the practice has committed to adopting Guided Care.

b. Explain the practice's rationale for adopting Guided Care.

c. Acknowledge that change is difficult and slow, but highlight the benefits of such a change in the long run.

d. Confirm that attendees have received a written description of Guided Care.

2. How Guided Care will work in the practice

a. Explain sources of funding.

b. Describe plans for hiring the nurse(s), identifying eligible patients, communicating with patients, and equipping office space.

c. Outline plans for orienting the nurse and holding nurse-staff meetings.

3. Questions and discussion

Physicians are involved in hiring, orienting, and evaluating the nurse, and are responsible for communicating regularly with the nurse about their patients and their teamwork. See Table 21-1 for a summary of the physicians' roles and responsibilities.

2. Identifying Patients

The 20% to 25% of patients on the physician's panel who have the highest estimated need for complex health care in the future are selected for Guided Care. This selection is accomplished by analyzing older patients' previous 12 months of health insurance claims with the Hierarchical Condition Category predictive model, which is available in the public domain. No high-risk patients are excluded because of a condition. Although clinicians are capable of identifying patients with multimorbidity, electronic predictive models can identify such patients more objectively, consistently, and efficiently.

3. Hiring the Nurse

The next step is to hire a registered nurse who has completed an accredited course (www.ijhn.jhmi.edu) and earned a Certificate in Guided Care Nursing. To attract strong applicants, the practice should offer a salary that is competitive with local hospital and home health care employers. See Box 21-1 for required and desirable qualities of Guided Care nurse applicants. See Box 21-2 for a sample job description.

TABLE 21-1 Physician's Role and Responsibilities in Guided Care

Task	Responsibility
Nurse selection	Each physician with whom the nurse will work reviews resumes, conducts interviews, and participates in the ranking of applicants.
Nurse orientation	Each physician meets with the nurse several times during the nurse's orientation to define how they will work together to care for patients. The physicians also introduce the Guided Care patients to the nurse during routine office visits and allow the nurse to observe the physician's style of interacting with these patients and their caregivers.
Building the caseload	The physician meets with the nurse for 20 to 25 minutes per patient to discuss and revise the Preliminary Care Guide that the nurse creates after the initial home assessment.
Ongoing Guided Care	The physician notifies the nurse of changes in their mutual patients' clinical status, especially admission to hospitals and emergency departments and referrals to specialists. The physician also replies to the nurse's messages about their patients' clinical conditions. To optimize their working relationship, the physician and the nurse meet periodically to give each other feedback and to refine their pattern of communication and collaboration. The physician also participates in the practice's periodic evaluation of the nurse's performance.

From Boult et al.[5]

4. Integrating the Nurse Into the Practice

A practice leader is responsible for orienting the nurse to the people and procedures of the practice, and for orienting the physicians and other staff members to the nurse and to the operational details of how Guided Care will work in the practice. The goals of the orientation are for the nurse to begin to develop effective teamwork with the physicians and

Box 21-1 Required and Desirable Qualities of Guided Care Nurse Applicants

The minimum requirements for people who apply for the Guided Care nurse position are as follows:

➤ Current licensure as a registered nurse

➤ Completion of an accredited, online course in Guided Care Nursing. For information on the course, please visit www.ijhn.jhmi.edu (look for Guided Care Nursing under the "Upcoming Programs" menu). This course could be completed between a nurse's hiring and starting to work in a Guided Care practice

➤ A Certificate in Guided Care Nursing issued by the American Nurses Credentialing Center. To earn the certificate, a nurse must successfully complete the Guided Care Nursing online course. The certificate could be earned between a nurse's hiring and starting to work in a Guided Care practice

➤ A minimum of 3 years of nursing experience, preferably with older patients

➤ Skill in using computers, the Internet, and health information technology

➤ Ability to travel frequently to hospitals, skilled nursing facilities, patients' homes, and other sites where patients receive care (as indicated by patients' needs)

Highly desirable qualities include the following:

➤ Excellent interpersonal skills

➤ Flexible and creative problem-solving skills

➤ Good clinical judgment and decision-making skills

➤ Demonstrated ability to work independently and as a member of an interdisciplinary team

➤ Clear understanding of the role of a Guided Care nurse

➤ Desire to learn and practice all of the position's components

➤ Commitment to "coaching" (rather than "teaching") patients to improve their health behaviors to attain their health-related goals

➤ Commitment to learning about and referring patients to health-related services in the local community

➤ Effective oral and written communication skills, and listening and assertion skills

Box 21-2 Sample Guided Care Nurse Job Description

POSITION TITLE: GUIDED CARE NURSE

Purpose:

To manage all aspects of patient-centered Guided Care for 50 to 60 frail elderly patients, working with one health care team. The nurse directly interfaces with physicians, health care teams, patients, and their unpaid caregivers in managing patient care.

Accountabilities:

The ideal candidate will possess excellent interpersonal skills, with a flexible and creative approach to problem solving. The candidate will have a demonstrated ability to work effectively as a member of an interdisciplinary team, displaying good clinical judgment and decision-making skills. As a team member, the Guided Care nurse must possess excellent communication skills, both written and verbal, and an ability to listen and be assertive, as required. Central to the role of the Guided Care nurse is a commitment to "coaching" (rather than "teaching") patients to improve their health behaviors to attain their health-related goals. An ability to work independently is essential.

The Guided Care nurse will have a clear understanding of the role and will demonstrate a commitment to implementation of the following accountabilities:

1. Comprehensive case management and care coordination for 50 to 60 frail elderly patients according to Guided Care principles. The Guided Care nurse is expected to provide the following services to each patient:

    a. Comprehensive geriatric home assessment

    b. Development and communication (with patient, caregiver, and primary care physician/health care team) of a comprehensive care plan based on evidence-based best practice for chronic illness

    c. Proactive management and follow-up (home visits and by telephone) according to care plan

    d. Management and coordination of all transitions in care:

        i. Communicate care plan to all providers in all setting of care (emergency departments, hospital, rehabilitation facility, nursing home, home care, and specialist)

        ii. Ensure that relevant providers receive timely clinical data for care treatment decisions in all settings of care (emergency departments, hospital, rehabilitation facility, nursing home, home care, and specialty care)

    e. Direct caregiver support, including ad hoc telephone advice

(continued)

> **Box 21-2** *(continued)*

> f. Facilitation of patient and caregiver access to community resources relevant to patient's needs, including referrals to transportation programs, Meals on Wheels, senior centers, chore services
>
> g. Incorporation of self-care and shared decision making in all aspects of patient care
>
> **Minimum requirements:**
>
> ➤ Current licensure as a registered nurse in the state where the practice is located and where the practice's patients live
>
> ➤ Completion of an accredited course in Guided Care nursing
>
> ➤ A Certificate in Guided Care Nursing issued by the American Nurses Credentialing Center
>
> ➤ Three years of nursing experience, preferably with older patients
>
> ➤ Proficiency in computer use, the Internet, and health information technology
>
> ➤ Ability to travel frequently to hospitals, skilled nursing facilities, patients' homes, and other sites where patients receive care (as indicated by patients' needs)
>
> From Boult et al.[5]

staff members, as well as to become familiar with office procedures and health-related resources in the local community. See Table 21-2 for the Guided Care Orientation Checklist.

TABLE 21-2 Guided Care Nurse Orientation Checklist

Date Completed	Supervisor's and Nurse's Initials	Orientation Topic
		Developing effective teamwork with physicians
		➤ First one-on-one orientation meeting with each physician
		➤ Nurse observation of each physician's interactions with Guided Care patients during office visits

➤ Each physician's observation of the nurse's interactions with Guided Care patients

➤ Second one-on-one orientation meeting with each physician

➤ Planning for periodic one-on-one physician meetings to improve teamwork

Developing effective teamwork with members of the office staff

The nurse acquires an understanding of:

➤ The roles of each member of the office staff

➤ The administrative relationships among all personnel

➤ The practice's processes for:

  ➤ Refilling prescriptions

  ➤ Arranging referrals

  ➤ Scheduling patients' appointments

  ➤ Reminding patients of appointments

  ➤ Notifying patients of test results

  ➤ Maintaining medical records (paper and electronic)

  ➤ Patient flow through the office

  ➤ Handling telephone messages

  ➤ Communicating with specific local hospitals and emergency departments about patients' admissions, discharges, and test results

  ➤ Contacting specific local health care professionals who often serve Guided Care patients: consultants, social workers, dieticians, pharmacists, health educators, rehabilitation and skilled nursing facilities, home care agencies, and hospice

  ➤ Providing after-hours on-call services

(continued)

TABLE 21-2 *(continued)*

Date Completed	Supervisor's and Nurse's Initials	Orientation Topic
		➤ Collecting copayments from patients
		➤ Submitting claims to insurance companies
		➤ Staff meetings and social events
		➤ Personnel policies: paychecks, employee benefits, vacations, sick time, reimbursement for expenses, parking, identification badges, security of the office building
		Completing necessary training in:
		➤ The use of the health information technology that supports Guided Care
		➤ Health Insurance Portability and Accountability Act (HIPAA)
		➤ Performance of relevant clinical functions within the practice: scheduling appointments, refilling prescriptions, and making referrals
		Creating an information database of community resources that serve Guided Care patients and caregivers
		➤ Area Agency on Aging, Meals on Wheels, senior centers, transportation programs, chore services, adult day health care centers, Alzheimer's Association, support groups, exercise programs, chronic disease self-management programs

From Boult et al.[5]

To begin building the essential nurse-physician teamwork, it is important that the nurse meet with each physician to define the many processes that they will soon conduct as a team (Table 21-3). To build teamwork as a new member of the office staff, the nurse meets with office staff to learn each person's role and the administrative relationships among them.

TABLE 21-3 Nurse-Physician Teamwork Activities

Category	Activities
Updating each other about the status of patients	➤ The Guided Care nurse provides the physician with a current list of their mutual Guided Care patients.
	➤ The Guided Care nurse notifies the physician of significant changes in their mutual patients' status, especially changes occurring between office visits and during care in hospitals and skilled nursing facilities.
	➤ The physician notifies the nurse of changes in their mutual patients' status, especially admissions to hospitals, visits to emergency departments, and referrals to specialists.
	➤ Depending on personal preferences, notifications could occur by e-mail, voice mail, hard copy notes, direct conversations, and/or entries in the medical record.
Providing care collaboratively	➤ The Guided Care nurse and physician discuss and modify the Preliminary Care Guides of patients who enroll in Guided Care.
	➤ The nurse joins the physician in the examining room during office visits, especially with patients who have acute problems or difficulty with communication, cognition, and/or adherence, or who have recently received care in hospitals or emergency departments.
Quality improvement processes	➤ The Guided Care nurse and the physician discuss ways to improve their Guided Care teamwork, and the nurse attends appropriate office staff meetings.

From Boult et al.[5]

The Guided Care nurse also begins to establish an individual, comprehensive plan for each of the 50 to 60 chronically ill patients of the practice who are eligible to receive Guided Care. The process usually requires 3 to 4 weeks to complete for each patient; see Table 21-4 for details.

5. Managing Guided Care

The success of Guided Care depends heavily on the physician's cooperation with the nurse and the nurse's consistent performance of certain essential activities. To ensure consistent performance of essential activities, the practice should operate a system of continuous quality improvement. The Guided Care nurse's

TABLE 21-4 Steps for Establishing a Comprehensive Plan for Each Guided Care Patient

Step	Action
1. Letter to patient	The practice administrator mails a letter to one or two eligible patients each week (with a copy sent to the nurse), notifying them that they are eligible (but not required) to receive Guided Care and that the practice's Guided Care nurse will call them within the next week.
2. Call to patient	The Guided Care nurse calls one or two eligible patients per week to provide more details about Guided Care, to answer their questions, to ask whether they are interested in receiving Guided Care, and, if appropriate, to schedule a time to visit their homes to assess their health status. For patients who are interested, the nurse uses pages 1–2 of the Health History Form to perform a focused brief review of the patient's medical record at the practice. The patient's chronic conditions determine what physical findings and laboratory results the nurse seeks and records on condition-specific assessment forms.
3. Consent	The Guided Care nurse visits each interested patient's home to meet the patient, describe Guided Care, answer the patient's questions, invite the patient to accept Guided Care and, if appropriate, obtain the patient's signature on a consent and authorization for the release of medical information form.
4. Initial assessment of the patient	After the patient signs the consent form, the nurse proceeds in conducting a comprehensive in-home assessment of the patient. For about 2 hours, the nurse follows pages 3–10 of the Health History Form in completing an in-depth interview with the patient and an evaluation of the safety and functionality of the patient's home environment.

5. Initial assessment of the caregiver	If, in the health history, the patient reports having a disability and identifies a family caregiver (or friend), the Guided Care nurse invites the caregiver by telephone to participate in the Guided Care education and support program for caregivers. If the caregiver accepts, the nurse sends the caregiver a confirming letter with an attached information form that the caregiver completes independently. The nurse then discusses the information on the form with the caregiver during a structured 30-minute assessment at a prearranged time and place, often the patient's home but sometimes by telephone at the caregiver's request. Sometimes these caregiver assessments can be completed immediately after the nurse's initial home assessment of the patient, if the caregiver is present and available.
6. Preliminary Care Guide	The nurse enters the patient assessment data collected from the home visit and from the patient's medical record into the practice's health information technology system and then generates a personalized, evidence-based, comprehensive Preliminary Care Guide.
7. Care Guide	The nurse and the patient's primary care physician meet for 20 to 25 minutes to review and modify the Preliminary Care Guide to create a Care Guide that reflects not only the applicable evidence-based guidelines for managing the patient's chronic conditions, but also the patient's life expectancy, comorbidity, and stated preferences for health care and health-related behaviors.
8. Revision of the Care Guide	The nurse discusses the Care Guide with the patient and caregiver and then revises it to make it consistent with the patient's intentions and capabilities—and to ensure that the patient and caregiver regard it as *their* plan. The nurse places the Care Guide in the medical record and uses it to communicate the plan for managing the patient's chronic conditions to each health care professional who treats the patient.
9. Creation of the patient's Action Plan	The nurse converts the Care Guide into a patient-friendly Action Plan, which expresses each desired action, such as taking medications and observing dietary restrictions, in the patient's language and in large print. The patient or caregiver displays the Action Plan prominently in a plastic jacket on the patient's refrigerator or cupboard, where it serves as a list of reminders of behaviors that will maximize the patient's health. The nurse also places a Guided Care identification card with the Medicare or other health insurance card in the patient's wallet to alert health care providers to the availability of the nurse to provide them with the patient's clinical information and to help coordinate their care with that of other providers.

supervisor should provide the nurse with a list of essential activities, a performance goal for each activity, a description of how the nurse should document each activity, and a schedule of quarterly feedback and evaluation meetings. The supervisor should also continue to manage the ongoing processes of Guided Care (see Box 21-3).

Technical Assistance in Adopting Guided Care

Several forms of technical assistance are available (www.medhomeinfo.org) to practices that wish to adopt the Guided Care model.

➤ An implementation manual titled *Guided Care: A New Nurse-Physician Partnership in Chronic Care* provides many tools, resources, and lessons learned for adopting Guided Care.[6]

➤ An accredited, online course in Guided Care nursing is a 6-week, 40-hour Web-based course and examination that leads to the American Nurses Credentialing Center's Certificate in Guided Care Nursing.

➤ An accredited, asynchronous, online, continuing medical education–eligible, nine-module course provides physicians, practice administrators, and other practice leaders with an awareness of the competencies that facilitate effective practice within all types of medical homes.

➤ Guidance in selecting health information technology is also available.

Box 21-3 Ongoing Processes of Guided Care That Supervisor Should Manage

➤ Communication with insurance organizations (eg, Medicare) that reimburse the practice for the costs of providing Guided Care for eligible patients

➤ Communication with eligible patients and caregivers regarding the administrative aspects of their eligibility and enrollment in the practice's Guided Care program

➤ Communication with the primary care physicians and the office staff regarding the ongoing operation and results of Guided Care within the practice

➤ Communication with and supervision of the Guided Care nurse. The supervisor should meet with the Guided Care nurse regularly to (a) assess and help improve the nurse's relationships and teamwork with the practice's physicians, office staff members, patients, and caregivers, and (b) discuss the feedback reports regarding the nurse's attainment of the preestablished performance goals, both recently and over time. To create these reports, the supervisor must monitor the nurse's documentation of these activities

TAKE-HOME POINTS

➤ Guided Care is a practical, interdisciplinary model of health care designed to improve the quality of life and efficiency of resource use for persons with medically complex health conditions. The role of the Guided Care nurse is to work in partnership with the primary care physician, the patient, the patient's caregiver, members of the office staff, and all other involved health care providers to attain the goals of Guided Care.

➤ Guided Care can be fully implemented in 6 to 9 months.

➤ Technical assistance is available to practices that wish to adopt Guided Care.

ACKNOWLEDGMENTS

We acknowledge Springer Publishing Company for their generosity in allowing some of the information from the book *Guided Care: A New Nurse-Physician Partnership in Chronic Care*[5] to be summarized in this chapter. We also acknowledge the following organizations and government agencies that provided support for our randomized controlled trial of Guided Care: the John A. Hartford Foundation, the Agency for Healthcare Research and Quality, the National Institute on Aging, and the Jacob and Valeria Langeloth Foundation.

REFERENCES

1. Boyd C. Guided Care: the clinical model. *Gerontologist.* 2007;47(1):S649.

2. Boult C, Reider L, Frey K, et al. Early effects of "Guided Care" on the quality of health care for multimorbid older persons: a cluster-randomized controlled trial. *J Gerontol A Biol Sci Med Sci.* 2008;63A(3):321–327.

3. Wolff JL, Rand-Giovannetti E, Palmer S, et al. Caregiving and chronic care: the Guided Care program for families and friends. *J Gerontol A Biol Sci Med Sci.* 2009;64A(7):785–791.

4. Leff B, Reider L, Frick KD, et al. Guided Care and the cost of complex health care: a preliminary report. *Am J Manag Care.* 2009;15(8):555–559.

5. Boult C, Giddens J, Frey K, Reider L, Novak T. *Guided Care: A New Nurse-Physician Partnership in Chronic Care.* New York, NY: Springer Publishing Co; 2009. www.springerpub.com/guidedcare. Accessed November 13, 2009.

CHAPTER | TWENTY-TWO

Program of All-Inclusive Care for the Elderly (PACE)

Matthew McNabney, MD

CASE

You are taking care of an 85-year-old woman who lives with her daughter. She has significant dementia of the Alzheimer type as well as advanced chronic obstructive pulmonary disease and coronary artery disease. She also suffers from periods of severe anxiety. She takes eight medications.

Although her daughter is committed to keeping her at home, this is becoming increasingly difficult. The patient is no longer able to perform her activities of daily living without supervision and assistance. She has shown a tendency to wander but has not become lost. In addition, her dementia and anxiety have made it very difficult to interpret her symptoms (chest/abdominal pain, dyspnea), and she has therefore been evaluated in the emergency department many times in the past few months.

As you consider the increasing care burden placed on the daughter and the inefficient use of the health care system, you decide to counsel the daughter on programs that might optimize this situation and allow the patient to remain living at home and avoid nursing home placement. She has Medicare, and your social worker has determined that her financial situation would make her eligible for Medicaid. You refer the patient and daughter to the local Program of All-inclusive Care for the Elderly (PACE) that provides services in her area.

OPPORTUNITIES

PACE is centered around the belief that it is better for the well-being of seniors with chronic care needs and their families to be served in the community whenever possible.

Eligibility requirements for PACE are as follows:

➤ Age 55 years or older

➤ Certified by state to need nursing home care

➤ Able to live safely in the community at the time of enrollment

➤ Living in a PACE service area (prescribed number of zip codes)

Although all participants must be certified to need nursing home care to enroll in PACE, only about 7% of PACE participants nationally reside in a nursing home. If a PACE enrollee does need nursing home care, the PACE program pays for it and continues to coordinate the enrollee's care.

PACE is a model of care that is designed to coordinate care by utilizing a highly integrated interdisciplinary care team. By using an adult day center as the "hub" of service, the PACE team addresses all aspects of care across the entire health care continuum.

PACE is a capitated program ("managed care"). The primary sources of these capitated funds are Medicare and Medicaid. For those who are not poor enough to qualify for Medicaid, it is possible to enroll in PACE through "private pay" (to cover the Medicaid portion). With these capitated funds, PACE programs are responsible for covering all health care costs (including hospital and physician charges).

The services offered through PACE are extensive. All standard Medicare benefits are provided as well as many that are not typically covered (such as hearing aids, dentures, and maintenance rehabilitation services). Individualized care plans are created by the PACE team, ideally with the input and participation of the enrollee and family. These care plans are updated by routine interdisciplinary team assessments.

Medical care is highly integrated into the team process, and medical decisions are heavily influenced by the team's assessments and recommendations. The medical providers provide all primary care. In fact, enrollees must transition their primary medical care to the PACE medical providers at the time of enrollment. (Although a few programs do allow community-based physicians to continue as primary care physicians, these are the exception.)

Although scheduled days at the PACE center are certainly focused on socialization and recreational activities, there are several other very important benefits. Through frequent observations by many members of the PACE team, the medical providers are made aware of issues that are pertinent to good medical care.

Because the medical offices/clinics are typically on-site with the PACE day centers, efficient medical evaluations can be readily performed.

CASE CONTINUED

When you discuss this option with your patient and her daughter, they are very interested. You make a referral to the PACE program intake coordinator. The patient is scheduled for an evaluation to establish eligibility and appropriateness for the program. You explain to the daughter that eligibility criteria are fairly strict to ensure that this program is reserved for those older adults with the greatest needs (nursing home eligible). Once the patient is enrolled in PACE, she transitions her primary care to the PACE providers and begins attending the PACE center 3 days per week (a typical number of days attended by enrollees). The daughter is able to regain some personal time, and she receives valuable feedback and guidance from the PACE team regarding care for her mother in the home. As a result of this support and the frequent medical assessments, her trips to emergency department are markedly reduced (only one in the next 6 months) and caregiver strain begins to ease.

BARRIERS

Older Adults Who Are Not Eligible

➤ Because PACE has specified eligibility criteria, many patients/family members can be disappointed to hear that they are not eligible.

➤ Many people who would theoretically benefit from PACE services are not yet impaired enough to meet the "nursing home eligible" criterion. For these individuals, it is important to explain why this criterion exists (to ensure appropriate allocation of costly services) and to educate them on the importance of continuous reassessment of increasing care needs and future referral to PACE.

➤ Some older adults will definitely meet the "nursing home eligible" criterion but are not able to be managed "safely in the community" (after assessment by the PACE team). For those people who have a strong desire to continue living at home, this can be very difficult to hear and process. However, PACE programs cannot enter into care arrangements when the program determines that it would remain unsafe for the patient even after implementation of PACE services.

➤ PACE programs are allowed to provide care to only those living in specified service areas. However, many older adults who live outside these areas may desire PACE services. Unless the individual relocates into the service area, enrollment is not allowed. This confinement to a service area is necessary but is an important limitation of PACE.

Limited Access to PACE

➤ Although the number of PACE programs in the United States is growing, this rate of growth is behind the projected need. Many areas could benefit from PACE that do not currently have such programs. There are some explanations for this, including:

  ➤ Geography/population density (Rural PACE initiative)

  ➤ Startup costs/capital

  ➤ Staffing challenges

  ➤ Degree of support from state (and federal) programs to facilitate expansion

SOLUTIONS

➤ *Refer* appropriate patients to an existing PACE program. Practitioners can become aware of PACE availability in the region (www.npaonline .org) and constantly think about those older patients who would be appropriate referrals.

➤ *Consider* PACE startup in your region. Where no PACE sites exist, practitioners, providers, and health systems can explore the possibility of starting a new PACE program. Although there are several steps and considerable costs to this venture, it is very realistic and leads to a very fulfilling and cutting-edge innovation in health care coordination for this population with complex needs.

➤ *Support* local and state initiatives for PACE expansion. You might be aware of efforts to start new PACE programs or expand existing PACE programs. You can play an important role in promoting innovative solutions to long-term care by advocating for these efforts.

➤ *Partner* with local and state officials on other (non-PACE) community-based long-term care solutions. Maintain an awareness of your state's rebalancing of long-term care expenditures toward community-based programs. Play a role in how those efforts are prioritized.

TAKE-HOME POINTS

➤ PACE is an established and respected care coordination model. It specifically serves the population of older adults who are nursing home eligible.

➤ PACE is an excellent example of team-coordinated care.

➤ Integrated financing (Medicare and Medicaid) allows for seamless care coordination along the continuum of acute and long-term care.

➤ PACE needs to expand at a faster rate in the United States to provide services to the growing number of older adults who are frail and chronically ill.

➤ Other non-PACE community-based long-term care programs are also developing and should be evaluated as potential options in the increasing efforts to shift long-term care to the community setting.

USEFUL RESOURCES

For general information on PACE, including regulations and startup guidelines (www.npaonline.org).

For information on team training, especially in rural areas (www.npaonline.org/Website/download.asp?id=2053).

For information from the Centers for Medicare and Medicaid Services regarding PACE and federal regulations, information on state agencies, list of PACE provider organizations, and provider application (www.cms.hhs.gov/PACE).

REFERENCE

Eng C, Pedulla J, Eleazer GP, McCann R, Fox N. Program of All-inclusive Care for the Elderly (PACE): an innovative model of integrated geriatric care and financing. *J Am Geriatr Soc.* 1997;45(2):223–232.

CHAPTER TWENTY-THREE

Basics of the Patient-Centered Medical Home

Beata Skudlarska, MD, CMD

James Judge, MD

CONSIDERING THE PATIENT-CENTERED MEDICAL HOME

You have recently joined a thriving multispecialty practice as a sixth primary care physician (PCP). Your practice serves many patients with complex medical conditions. Your group has just been approached by a forward-thinking insurance consortium to volunteer for a patient-centered medical home (PCMH) demonstration project. This particular payer is willing to add on substantial bonuses for practices fulfilling National Committee for Quality Assurance (NCQA) level 2 and 3 standards for PCMH. Your state medical society is also interested in working with your practice to solicit more contracts from other insurers and employers. You are put in charge of presenting the concepts of PCMH to the senior partners of your practice. Your group is highly respected for providing excellent care, and you see PCMH as an opportunity to be rewarded for the quality service you already provide.

You want to provide care that is best for your patients, but you don't really understand what a "medical home" is all about and what a practice must do to qualify for this designation. You also don't know how this will benefit your practice from the standpoint of quality and reimbursement.

OPPORTUNITIES

The term *medical home* was first introduced in 1967 by the American Academy of Pediatrics and is centered on the concept of a continuous relationship with a personal physician. This physician coordinates care for both wellness and illness. Other cornerstones of the medical home include accountability, access to information, expanded service hours, and evidence-based medical decision making. It is crucial to realize that PCMH is much more than management of chronic diseases and is especially adaptable to good geriatric care.

In 2007, the American Academy of Family Physicians (AAFP), American Academy of Pediatrics (AAP), American College of Physicians (ACP), and American Osteopathic Association (AOA) issued a statement of the seven core principles of the PCMH.[1] These principles are as follows, along with opportunities to improve care:

1. *Personal physician:* "each patient has an ongoing relationship with a personal physician trained to provide first contact, continuous and comprehensive care."

2. *Physician-directed medical practice:* "the personal physician leads a *team* [emphasis added] of individuals at the practice level who collectively take responsibility for the ongoing care of patients."

   ➤ Team members can include medical assistants, nurses, nurse practitioners, physician assistants, social workers, pharmacists, office assistants, or any other office staff member who contributes to the care of patients.

   ➤ Although physicians may work with all members in practice, clearly defined roles and process of care coordination will contribute to efficient utilization of all team members' skill sets.

   ➤ Chapters 20 to 22 describe additional models of care that emphasize care coordination, which is the basis of excellent care for older adults or those with complex medical needs.

3. *Whole-person orientation:* "the personal physician is responsible for providing for all the patient's health care needs or taking responsibility for appropriately arranging care with other qualified professionals."

   ➤ This can provide an opportunity to improve collaboration within a specialty group or community.

   ➤ Subspecialty members may initially feel uneasy about the concept of PCMH and fear decreased access of patients to their care and possible financial implications to their practice. However, clear communication regarding goals and expectations should mitigate such concerns.

4. *Coordination of care:* "Care is coordinated and/or integrated across all elements of the complex health care system . . . and the patient's community . . . . Care is facilitated by registries, information technology, health information exchange and other means to assure that patients get the indicated care when and where they need and want it in a culturally and linguistically appropriate manner."

➤ In addition to coordinating daily care, care transitions across settings (emergency department, hospital, rehabilitation facility, skilled nursing, etc) can be improved. See Chapter 28 for more details on transitions of care.

➤ Additionally, relationships with community nursing, home care, and hospice can be strengthened to increase services for your patient base.

➤ Patient information materials should be available in multiple languages. Chapter 6 addresses patient education forms and Chapter 32 considers culturally effective care.

5. *Quality and safety:* "Quality and safety are hallmarks of the medical home:

➤ Practices advocate for their patients to support the attainment of optimal, patient-centered outcomes that are defined by a care planning process driven by a compassionate, robust partnership between physicians, patients, and the patient's family.

➤ Evidence-based medicine and clinical decision-support tools guide decision making.

➤ Physicians in the practice accept accountability for continuous quality improvement through voluntary engagement in performance measurement and improvement.

➤ Patients actively participate in decision-making and feedback is sought to ensure patients' expectations are being met.

➤ Information technology is utilized appropriately to support optimal patient care, performance measurement, patient education, and enhanced communication.

➤ Practices go through a voluntary recognition process by an appropriate non-governmental entity to demonstrate that they have the capabilities to provide patient-centered services consistent with the medical home model.

➤ Patients and families participate in quality improvement activities at the practice level."

6. *Access to care:* "Enhanced access to care is available through systems such as open scheduling, expanded hours and new options for communication between patients, their personal physician, and practice staff."

➤ Consider ways to accommodate open access for your practice. Modified scheduling may be required for practices with large numbers of older adults (see Chapter 16 for help on managing scheduling complexities).

➤ Extended hours may improve access, but consider polling patients or piloting hours before full implementation.

➤ E-mailing patients and/or their families can facilitate access and communication.

➤ To continue the scenario presented at the beginning of the chapter, let's say the local hospital your practice uses most of the time has recently offered to electronically transmit discharge summaries and emergency department visit records to your group.

7. *Payment:* "Payment appropriately recognizes the added value provided to patients who have a patient-centered medical home." In our scenario, three major ways of payment are being considered:

➤ Enhanced fee-for-service for achieving PCMH status

➤ Care management fee (dollar amount per patient per month; the amount may vary with complexity of patients' needs)

➤ Shared savings concepts

It is clear that whatever payment structure develops will be outcome-based and the concept of accountable care will be at its center. Practices should ensure that any financial arrangements offered by insurers justify additional efforts put in place in order to acquire the NCQA certification or to implement required practice changes.

CHALLENGES

Particular obstacles need to be considered in order for your practice to succeed with transformation to a PCMH. They represent common issues faced by many provider groups:

➤ *No consensus on the details that make a medical home.* While many insurance companies and pilot programs use NCQA certification to define the basic characteristics required to be recognized as a PCMH, other interpretations of how best to implement the seven principles can hinder attempts to change.

➤ *High-speed, high-volume care provided by most primary care practices.* This often makes physicians reluctant to engage in new, time-consuming initiatives unless benefits of these initiatives are clear and desirable to physicians and other members of the practice.

➤ *A tradition of PCPs having little respect in multispecialty practices, or within many health systems.* You will need to restore the central role of the PCP. In a recent study 70% of patients were unable to identify their PCP by name, and of the remaining 30% who thought they could, 40%

were wrong. Hopefully that is not true for your practice. The PCP will be responsible for coordinating the care for the patient, based on an understanding of the big picture and the patients' values and goals of care.

➤ *Inefficiency.* You and most of the members of your practice may not be working at your fullest potential. In your practice, just like in many others, nurses often do office assistant jobs, nurse practitioners do nurses' jobs, and physicians spend time engaging in activities that can be delegated to the nurse practitioners and nurses. Critical assessment of the processes in the practice including written protocols may be necessary to eliminate these patterns of behavior.

➤ *Patients with complex needs requiring a longer time during the visits.* They may not always understand and follow visit instructions. Identifying patients whose medical needs are particularly complex and who visit the practice often is essential. The focus is to have all information from the extended clinical team (home care, laboratory, consultations, and caregivers) available at the time of the visit. This permits the physician or physician extender to be efficient and effective during the visit to adjust plans of care and coordinate care better.

➤ *Cost and logistics of changes.* System redesign to prohibit duplication of orders, tests, and services may be complicated or expensive to implement.

➤ *Difficulty in using evidence-based medicine to guide the process of care for certain populations.* Healthcare Effectiveness Data and Information Set (HEDIS) measures may conflict with good care of older adults with multiple conditions and advanced diseases. Disease treatment guidelines developed for adults with a single condition should not be applied without review of the overall disease burden of your elderly patients. The risk and burdens of treatment vs the benefit that your patient is likely to experience must be soberly assessed. Following guidelines, particularly in diabetes mellitus, may worsen quality of life for patients with advanced disease. The American Geriatrics Society Web site has useful tools, especially the guideline on diabetes mellitus (http://www.americangeriatrics.org/files/documents/JAGSfinal05.pdf). Discussions with patients and their families regarding *goals of care* must be clearly documented. This often requires retraining of the physicians who may not be comfortable addressing issues of advanced diseases. It also may require longer visits with the physician and a nurse or care manager.

➤ *Need for information technology upgrades.* Seamless flow of information does depend on the quality of the electronic medical record (EMR) system, and graduating a practice into the PCMH model often requires a new information technology application. The ideal situation would include one system across the continuum of care, but this is not always attainable. Patient access to information is a separate challenge and may be addressed by e-mailing or mailing test and bloodwork results and reminders of visits, wellness examinations, and tests.

➤ *Ensuring complete information capture.* Capturing information on visits and orders executed outside the practice (other specialists, nursing homes, hospitals) is important for success of the program.

➤ *Ability to designate an RN to serve as a patient care manager, with full access to all patients' clinical records.* Some larger practices, employers, and larger plans are using centralized (out of the office) telephonic care manager systems.

➤ *Monitoring and analyzing care.* Many practices do not know how effective they are in immunization rates and capturing other elements of preventive care. Management of chronic diseases may need improvement, with clearly defined outcome measures. Goals of care discussions will need to become standard of care. Developing and utilizing a population disease registry will be required. All these adjustments will take time and effort of the whole practice team.

SOLUTIONS: PRACTICE CHANGES

1. Assess the existing resources in your practice. Most functioning internal medicine, pediatric, or family practice offices already follow many of the principles of the PCMH listed above. The EMR is the component most often missing.

2. Always keep the *goal* in mind. Consider how to build and sustain a strong personal relationship between each patient and his or her PCP.

3. Have all team members identify what they would like to spend more time doing and what they are spending too much time doing. This can identify both professional goals and opportunities for each staff member to work at his or her highest capacity. Simple reorganization and reassignment steps may be enough to optimize your practice team.

4. Identify the clinical information "black holes" in your care system and drill down to root cause(s). Don't stop at the first cause—keep drilling until you have successfully addressed the problem with long–term, sustainable solutions.

5. Structure your team decision-making processes and schedule:

   a. *Weekly:* planning meeting to anticipate upcoming needs and a care management meeting (once or twice weekly depending on usual need and complexity of patient population). Table 23-1 is a worksheet/checklist to help a PCMH prepare for the next week's visits and ensure that the tasks from the previous week were completed.

TABLE 23-1 Practice Tasks for a Visit by Visit Type

TYPE OF VISIT OR MANAGEMENT					
Elements of Care Process	Episodic	Preventive	Chronic Condition PCP Manages	Chronic Conditions With >1 Specialist	Advanced Illness, Hospice or Palliative Care
Previsit: obtain and assemble required information		X	X	X	X
Consultant notes/2-way communication			X	X	X
Diagnostic tests/ discharge summaries			X	X	X
Rehabilitation/therapies				X	X
Care manager tasks/ handoffs				X	X
Home care				X	X
Hospice team					X
Visit					
Acute history	X		X	X	Home visit may be needed
Examination	X	X	X	X	X
Diagnosis	X	X	X	X	X
Treatment	X	X	X	X	X
Lifestyle changes		X	X	X	X
Patient discussion		X	X	X	X
Family discussion		X	X	X	X
Goals of care discussion		X		X	X
Postvisit handoffs/tasks for medical home team and communication to other health care providers					
Rehabilitation/therapies				X	X
Care manager tasks/ handoffs				X	X
Home care				X	X
Hospice team					X

b. *Daily:* a brief team meeting at the beginning of the day to scan the tasks of the day to make each visit efficient and effective. Confirm that all diagnostic and consultation reports are in the chart or EMR for each visit.

c. *Daily:* Review tomorrow's schedule and assign tasks to ensure that all pending clinical information is available for the visit.

d. See Chapters 11 and 24 for additional resources related to team building and communication.

6. Sustain your transformation. The team care approach and buy-in from nonphysician members of the practice who will also share the benefits of the PCMH can be accomplished by one-on-one discussion, monthly update meetings, and rewards (financial and nonfinancial) for the most active members of the practice.

7. Don't reinvent the wheel. Review the tools for practice transformation that have been developed by American Academy of Family Practice and the American College of Physicians (links are listed in the Useful Resources section). There are other vendors as well.

8. Determine whether you wish to be recognized by the NCQA as a PCMH. Review the list of components of the medical home and consider how they can incorporate elements to improve care for older adults in the practice (Table 23-2). There are three levels of PCMH, which are determined by how many of the elements your practice has incorporated. The boldface elements in Table 23-2 are essential for recognition. Identify what you are doing very well, adequately, and poorly.

TABLE 23-2 Components of the Medical Home

NCQA Standards*	Geriatrics-Specific Details
1. Access and communication	
A. **Has written standards for patient access and patient communication**	Use of standardized patient materials in multiple languages for common conditions (incontinence, dementia, falls)
B. Uses data to show it meets its standards for patient access and communication	
2. Patient tracking and registry function	
A. Uses data system for basic patient information (mostly nonclinical data)	
B. Has clinical data system with clinical data in searchable data fields	

C. Uses the clinical data system	
D. **Uses paper or electronic-based charting tools to organize clinical information**	

E. **Uses data to identify important diagnoses and conditions in practice**	1. Identify high-risk/vulnerable elders
	
	2. Geriatric conditions:
	
	   a. Incontinence
	
	   b. Memory disorders/dementia
	
	   c. Falls risk
	
	   d. Functional status
	
	3. Polypharmacy (>6 medicines)

F. Generates lists of patients and reminds patients and clinicians of services needed (population management)	1. Influenza vaccine 2. Pneumovax 3. Diabetes mellitus quarterly tasks 4. Goals of care discussions for advanced illness

3. Care management

A. **Adopts and implements evidence-based guidelines for three conditions**	Geriatric conditions for which there are existing guidelines: 1. Incontinence 2. Memory disorders/dementia
	3. Falls risk/recurrent fallers 4. Polypharmacy See ACOVE 3 Web site for selection of other performance standards for vulnerable elders: www.rand.org/health/projects/acove/acove3
B. Generates reminders about preventive services for clinicians	
C. Uses nonphysician staff to manage patient care	Front desk alerts practitioners if: 1. Missed appointments, or patient shows up on wrong day, confusion on patient's or family's part with follow-up plans or medications; flag for cognitive testing

(continued)

TABLE 23-2 *(continued)*

NCQA Standards*	Geriatrics-Specific Details
	2. Track medication refills for patients flagged for adherence concerns
	3. Staff assesses logistical and financial barriers to medication adherence
	4. Proactive calls to other health care providers to drive the PCMH as managing the plan of care
	5. Proactive management of patients receiving home care services, with weekly update of physician
D. Conducts care management, including care plans, assessing progress addressing barriers	Schedule one or two sessions per week with medical home team with call-in hours for home care agencies and hospice
E. Coordinates care/follow-up for patients who receive care in inpatient and outpatient facilities	System to alert medical home when patient is admitted to hospital, coordinate care with hospitalist and discharge planner related to discharge and follow-up (skilled nursing facility and home care); track consultations to note when PCP needs to approve changes in plans of care
4. Patient self-management support	
A. Assesses language preference and other communication barriers	Includes assessment for hearing/vision/cognitive impairment as part of evaluation for communication barriers
B. **Actively supports patient self-management**	1. Supports "self-management" for patients with cognitive impairment by including family/caregivers 2. Discussion of goals of care before a crisis
5. Electronic prescribing	
A. Uses electronic system to write prescriptions	
B. Has electronic prescription writer with safety checks	
C. Has electronic prescription writer with cost checks	

6. Test tracking	
A. **Tracks tests and identifies abnormal results systematically**	
B. Uses electronic systems to order and retrieve tests and flag duplicate tests	
7. Referral tracking	
A. **Tracks referrals using paper-based or electronic system**	Essential element for complex patients; ensure that PCP notes are transmitted to consultants
8. Performance reporting and improvement	
A. **Measures clinical and/or service performance by physician or across the practice**	1. Hospital readmission rate 2. Percentage evaluated and adherence to guidelines for #3A 3. Percentage of patients with goals of care and advanced directives in medical record 4. Immunization rates 5. ACOVE 3 process measures appropriate for vulnerable elders www.rand.org/health/projects/acove/acove3
B. Survey of patients' care experience	Potential questions ➤ Does the patient or family member understand why they are taking each medicine? ➤ Does the MD and the medical home understand their goals of care? ➤ Does the office reply in a timely fashion to clinical questions?
C. **Reports performance across the practice or by physician**	
D. Sets goals and takes action to improve performance	
E. Produces reports using standardized measures	

(continued)

TABLE 23-2 *(continued)*

NCQA Standards*	Geriatrics-Specific Details
F. Transmits reports with standardized measures electronically to external entities	
9. Advanced electronic communications	
A. Availability of interactive Web site	
B. Electronic patient identification	
C. Electronic care management support	

*Essential elements are shown in boldface type.

9. Quality indicators, like the Acute Care for Elders (ACOVE) Project, can help guide decision-making tools and quality improvement initiatives within the context of the PCMH. (See the Useful Resources section.)

10. Do not let your lack of an EMR delay your practice transformation. However, an EMR is likely in your future and is essential for meeting higher-level accreditation as an NCQA PCMH. (See Chapter 27, The Electronic Medical Record (EMR): Considerations for Geriatric Care.)

11. Partner with your state medical society, local hospital, and/or large employers who are already interested in the principles of a PCMH. This may prove very helpful, especially in choosing an EMR that will be able to access diagnostic test results and hospital reports. Partnering may help you get involved in programs that will give your practice the additional revenue you deserve for your efforts and investment in practice transformation.

USEFUL RESOURCES

The following links are the leading sites to help you analyze your practice and develop a plan for practice transformation.

➤ AAFP, ACP, AAP, AOA. Joint Principles of the Patient-Centered Medical Home. March 2007 (www.medicalhomeinfo.org/joint%20Statement.pdf).

➤ TransforMED, a PCMH transformation toolkit from an independent subsidiary of the American Academy of Family Practice (http://transformed.com/index.cfm).

➤ Medical Home Builder, a PCMH transformation toolkit from the American College of Physicians (www.acponline.org/running_practice/pcmh/).

➤ NCQA standards: how to be certified as a PCMH (www.ncqa.org/tabid/631/Default.aspx).

➤ American Geriatrics Society

 ➤ Link to care principles and patient and caregiver materials for common conditions in your geriatric patients: memory loss, falls, depression, and incontinence (http://www.americangeriatrics.org/health_care_professionals/clinical_practice/ featured_programs_products/).

 ➤ Link to guidelines on diabetes mellitus, vertigo, syncope, and other conditions (http://www.americangeriatrics.org/health_care_professionals/clinical_practice/ clinical_guidelines_recommendations).

➤ ACOVE quality indicators

 ➤ (www.annals.org/content/135/8_Part_2/653.full). Accessed March 1, 2010.

 ➤ Shekelle PG, MacLean CH, Morton SC, et al. ACOVE quality indicators. *Ann Intern Med*. 2001;135(8 pt 2):653–667.

➤ Perspective on PCMH and accountable care organizations (for background and big picture). Rittenhouse DR, Shortell SM, Fisher ES. Primary care and accountable care—two essential elements of delivery-system reform. *N Engl J Med*. 2009;361(24):2301–2303. (http://content. nejm.org/cgi/content/full/NEJMp0909327v2).

REFERENCE

1. National Center for Medical Home Implementation. Joint Principles of the Patient-Centered Medical Home. March 2007. www.medicalhomeinfo.org/joint%20Statement.pdf.

CHAPTER TWENTY-FOUR

Effective Communication With an Office Team

Paul Mulhausan, MD, MHS

MRS APPLE'S EXPERIENCE

Mrs Apple is an 88-year-old widowed woman living alone in her home of 50 years. She presents for evaluation after a neighbor recently referred her to the Department of Human Services (DHS) for self-neglect. One week before her appointment with you, the DHS case worker calls you with questions regarding her lack of capacity and possible Alzheimer's disease. She was diagnosed with stage 1 breast cancer 2 years ago and has consistently chosen not to undergo lumpectomy or radiation therapy. Her other medical problems include hypertension, osteoarthritis, and generalized anxiety disorder. Her main goal is to stay at home.

OPPORTUNITIES

Physicians providing geriatric care face the difficult task of overseeing the care of patients across a complex set of needs and settings, along with a matrix of other health professionals. Geriatric care encompasses not only medical care, but social care, health promotion, and illness prevention. Coordinating this care, responding to multiple patient needs, and delivering care across settings requires effective communication across the disciplines that make up the office team.[1-4]

In Mrs Apple's case, there are numerous issues at play in her presentation:

➤ What is the role of her breast cancer?

➤ Is there an unrecognized cognitive deficit impacting her independence?

➤ Is there another unrecognized medical problem affecting her wellness and function?

➤ Does she remain capable of independent decision making?

➤ What services are needed to support her goal to live at home?

➤ What personal resources are available for her to support her present living arrangements in light of evolving dependency for activities of daily living and instrumental activities of daily living?

➤ What community resources are available to support her functional needs, and can they be implemented in her home?

➤ What are her family resources, and can they support her functional needs?

Evaluating Mrs Apple's present circumstances and then implementing an appropriate treatment plan that achieves her goals is best accomplished by working through the coordinated efforts of an interdisciplinary team. Along with the patient and caregiver, the core disciplines of the geriatric interdisciplinary team in the ambulatory practice setting are medicine, nursing, and social work. In many offices, the team is characterized by a patient and caregiver-physician-nurse partnership collaborating with an offsite social worker. In some settings, the team may be extended to include a pharmacy, visiting nurse, physical therapy, occupational therapy, speech therapy, and psychology.[3] Team members integrate their observations, fields of expertise, and areas of decision making to collaborate and coordinate with one another to optimize care.[4]

Skills for a Successful Office Team

For an office team to work successfully, its members must be proficient in six essential skills[3]:

➤ Communication

➤ Collaboration

➤ Coordination

➤ Brainstorming

➤ Joint decision making

➤ Team leadership

Of these skills, communication may be most critical, yet the most difficult to master. Current team theory suggests that teams will be most effective if all members engage actively in discussion to set the team's goals and methods.[5] *Effective team communication* predicts the sharing of accurate information, clear understanding of the team goals, the utilization of the specialized knowledge of team disciplines, resolution of misunderstandings, and feelings of trust and belonging among team members. *Poor team communication* can result in misunderstanding, poor interpersonal interactions among team members, inefficient use of time, and mistiming in the sequence of a treatment plan. This interdisciplinary communication is especially important in the care of older patients because their multifaceted health problems require greater contact with the health care system and more attention to the maintenance of function and quality of life.[6]

BARRIERS

Numerous barriers to effective interdisciplinary communication have been documented in the medical literature. Some of these are rooted in interpersonal communication styles, while others are rooted in culture, disciplinary tradition, and the complexity of a team's communication needs. Recognized barriers to effective communication among office teams include the following[7]:

➤ Team composition that is not appropriate for intended goals

➤ Language barriers

➤ Cultural barriers

➤ Absence of shared purpose

➤ Lack of training

➤ Leadership ambiguity

➤ Role ambiguity

➤ Excessively large team size

➤ Absence of mechanisms for the timely exchange of information

Differences in the philosophies of practice and professional training can also influence communication with team members from different disciplines who might see the same circumstances, but interpret the meaning differently. Each of the disciplines participating in the team has evolved independently, and each has its own tradition, culture, and regulatory environment. Individual members of the interdisciplinary team may have little understanding and, in some cases, respect for each other's roles.[8] These conceptual differences in approach to care that can exist across disciplines, known as "culture splits," may also present a barrier to effective communication.[9] Finally, scarce resources and time pressures represent major impediments to effective communication among team members. Perceived workload is frequently reported as a barrier, and scarce resources may limit organizational support for the team.

SOLUTIONS

Fundamental to the effective workings of an office team is a collaborative climate characterized by mutual respect and trust.[10,11] Without this collaborative climate, teams are at high risk for miscommunication and dysfunction. Team members must learn about other team members' expertise, background, knowledge, and values.[4] They must clarify and learn their individual roles and the processes required to work collaboratively. Interest and ability to work with other team members on an equal footing are crucial to effective teamwork. Although teamwork among health care disciplines can create hierarchy/egalitarian tension, many teams function well with a hierarchical structure as long as there is mutual respect.[8]

There is little empiric evidence to define the one best way for physicians to communicate most effectively with members of the office team. However, there are well-accepted communication techniques that facilitate the sharing of information, the formulation of team goals, and the achievement of those goals.[6]

Techniques to Foster Team Communication[6,9]

➤ Encourage communication and participation. Ask for input and feedback from all members of the team.

➤ Ask team members for their opinions and feelings to encourage discussion.

➤ Listen carefully to what the other team members are saying.

➤ Ask for a summary of the discussion.

➤ Paraphrase and reflect on what fellow team members say to ensure understanding.

➤ Ask for examples.

➤ Probe ideas in greater depth.

➤ When there is repetition or confusion, ask fellow team members for explanations.

Elements of an Ideal System for Interdisciplinary Communication[6,9]

Reasonable people can and do differ in their thoughts and ideas with each other. Diversity among team members enhances creativity. Once teams identify differences in opinions and the responses to them, the group will need to take action to resolve them. Successful resolution requires the ability to communicate effectively, as well as express thoughts and issues, while focusing on the search for win-win solutions. Again, there is no one recognized technique to manage or avoid team disagreement, but techniques have been described that have been proven effective to enhance team collaborations:

➤ Welcome the existence of differences of opinion, bring it into the open, and use it as potential for change.

➤ Establish built-in processes to review decisions.

➤ Examine overlapping team roles and renegotiation of role assignments.

➤ Separate the person from the problem to diffuse the emotional component of the disagreement by showing respect, listening carefully, and giving all parties the opportunity to express their views.

➤ Do not express opinions as fact.

➤ Provide justification for statements.

➤ Ask others for reasoning before offering a counter opinion.

➤ Clarify the nature of the disagreement as seen by both parties. Is this the real problem?

➤ Deal with one problem at a time, beginning with the easier issue.

➤ Listen with understanding rather than evaluation. Use the communication skills of listening, clarifying, and reflecting.

➤ Attack data, facts, assumptions, and conclusions, but not the individual.

➤ Identify areas of agreement. Focus on common interests, not positions.

➤ Brainstorm about possible solutions.

➤ Invent new solutions where both parties gain.

➤ Evaluate and review the problem-solving process after implementing the plan.

Regular team meetings are a well-recognized strategy to improve communication with the office team. Much essential communication among team members occurs outside of the meetings, but regular meetings of the office team can help to break down professional barriers and improve interprofessional communications. The improved communication may assist in the resolution of the issue and promote positive interpersonal relations. *Teams that meet regularly are generally found to achieve greater levels of innovation.*[6]

Many physicians find the time pressures of practice a barrier to convening regular team meetings. For a team to operate successfully, it needs organizational support, both for team working and for team members. Teams work within organizations and will be affected by interaction with the organization. If an organization agrees that team care is important, it must recognize the time that is required. The key elements of an ideal system for interdisciplinary communication have been proposed:

➤ A well-designed medical record system

➤ A regularly scheduled forum to discuss and evaluate team function and development

➤ A regularly scheduled forum for team members to discuss patient management issues

➤ A mechanism for communicating with the external system within which the team operates.

TAKE-HOME POINTS

➤ Effective team communication is essential to the successful delivery of interdisciplinary care.

➤ The barriers to effective team communication are many, but they can be overcome with a commitment to shared work and a climate of mutual respect.

➤ The communication skills that facilitate effective communication can be learned, practiced, and mastered.

➤ Techniques to minimize and resolve the issue(s) can be learned, practiced, and mastered.

➤ Successful team communication requires organizational support and commitment.

➤ The basic elements of an ideal system for interdisciplinary communication have been described and can be easily implemented when organizational commitment is in place.

USEFUL RESOURCES

American Geriatrics Society Geriatric Interdisciplinary Team Training (GITT) Kit

➤ This resource includes learning tools for team communication and consensus building (http://www.gittprogram.org/index.html).

John A. Hartford Foundation Inc GITT Geriatric Interdisciplinary Team Training Program

➤ This program includes resources for team assessment and products for team development and implementation (www.gittprogram.org).

REFERENCES

1. Williams BC, Reminton T, Foulk M. Teaching interdisciplinary geriatrics team care. *Acad Med.* 2002;77(9):935.

2. Keough ME, Field TS, Gurwitz JH. A model of community-based interdisciplinary team training. *Acad Med.* 2002;77(9):936.

3. Dyer CB, Hyer K, Feldt KS, et al. Frail older patient care by interdisciplinary teams: a primer for generalists. *Gerontol Geriatr Educ.* 2004;24(2):51–62.

4. Institute of Medicine Committee on the Health Professions Education Summit. Health professions education: a bridge to quality. Greiner AC, Knebel E, eds. Washington, DC: National Academy Press; 2003.

5. Carletta JC. Communication and effectiveness in primary health care teams. Workshop on Dependability in Healthcare Informatics, Edinburgh, Scotland, March 22–23, 2001. http://homepages.inf.ed.ac.uk/jeanc/DIRC-paper.pdf Accessed May 1, 2010.

6. Clark PG. Values in health care professional socialization: implications for geriatric education in interdisciplinary teamwork. *Gerontologist.* 1997;37(4):441–451.

7. John A. Hartford Foundation GITT Curriculum Guide. Topic 3: team communication and conflict resolution. American Geriatrics Society 2009. http://www.gittprogram.org/index.html. Accessed December 3, 2009.

8. Payne S, Kerr C, Hawker S, et al. The communication of information about older people between health and social care practitioners. *Age Aging.* 2002;31:107–117.

9. Reuben DB, Levy-Storms L, Yee MN, et al. Disciplinary split: a threat to geriatrics interdisciplinary team training. *JAGS.* 2004;52(6):1000–1006.

10. Williams BC, Remington TL, Foulk MA, Whall AL. Teaching interdisciplinary geriatrics ambulatory care: a case study. *Gerontol Geriatr Educ.* 2006;26(3):29–45.

11. Xyrichis A, Lowton K. What fosters or prevents interprofessional teamworking in primary and community care? *Int J Nursing Stud.* 2008;45:140–153.

CHAPTER TWENTY-FIVE

Coordination of Care With Nonphysician Geriatric Service Providers

Arline Bohannon, MD

Angela Gentili, MD

MR E. G.'S EXPERIENCE

Mr E. G. is a 78-year-old African American male who lives alone in subsidized senior housing. Mr E. G. has an eighth-grade education with limited health literacy. He has multiple medical problems that include chronic obstructive airway disease, coronary artery disease with ischemic cardiomyopathy (ejection fraction 35%), and type 2 diabetes mellitus (treated with oral hypoglycemic agents). During the past 6 months, Mr E. G. has had several admissions for exacerbations of congestive heart failure. The most recent admission was due to noncompliance; he did not resume furosemide therapy after spironolactone had been added to his medication regimen. He did not understand that he needed both diuretics.

INTRODUCTION

In a multidisciplinary collaborative practice, several steps can be taken to improve patient care and reduce emergency department and hospital admissions:

➤ *Shared visits between MD and nurse practitioner (NP):* Both the physician and other clinical providers are able to examine the patient and participate in the care plan.

➤ *Transitional care visits:* The NP makes home visits after discharge. At this visit, the plan of care is reviewed, medication reconciliation is completed, and any psychosocial barriers are identified.

➤ *NP as liaison:* NPs can facilitate communication between subspecialists and providers, patients, and caregivers.

➤ *Role of case manager:* Case manager helps coordinate care and other services.

OPPORTUNITIES

In addition to reducing unnecessary hospital admissions, care coordination with nonphysician providers can improve transitions and maximize the time spent with the primary care provider. To provide effective care coordination with nonphysician providers, it is essential to understand their potential roles and responsibilities.

Midlevel Providers

Midlevel providers such as geriatric nurse practitioners and physician assistants are clinicians who can diagnose and treat geriatric patients and who can practice in all settings—long-term care, outpatient, and inpatient. Shared visits in a hospital-based clinic are effective, as the physician is available for on-site consultation (see www.cms.hhs.gov for details on billing and documentation). These clinical providers can perform intensive geriatric case management in either the home or clinic setting, ensuring frequent follow-up to provide patient education and assessment of early disease exacerbation to prevent hospital admission or emergency department visits.

Geriatric Case Managers

Case managers are usually nurses, social workers, or psychologists with advanced training in gerontology who are able to help families provide care for frail elders. Geriatric case managers can assist with transitions from independent living to higher skill levels, and they can assist families in identifying community resources, eg, Meals on Wheels, adult day care, or transportation. Geriatric case managers may also accompany elders with limited family support to their physician appointments. Most geriatric care managers charge a fee for their services (www.caremanager.org).

Rehabilitation Services

Occupational, physical, and speech therapists are professionals who focus on maintaining or improving function in the elderly. Referrals for rehabilitation professionals can be obtained through home health agencies or local hospitals. Home evaluations by rehabilitation professionals are most helpful in identifying barriers that may prevent an elder from living independently, eg, safety hazards, cognitive impairment.

Geriatric Social Workers

These professionals can assist with identifying community resources available to elders. Depending on the type of license of the social worker, he/she can provide mental health assessment and counseling. Referrals for social work services can be obtained through the area department of aging, local hospital, or home health agencies.

Nursing Staff

The outpatient nursing staff effectively performs patient triage so that urgent problems can be identified expeditiously. Home health agency nursing staff provides assessment for patients who are homebound and find it difficult to comply with outpatient appointments. It is particularly helpful to those practitioners who do not make home visits as part of their practice.

Geriatric Pharmacist

Pharmacists with expertise in geriatric medication management can review medications for inappropriate drugs and drug interactions, review patients with five or more medications to minimize problems with polypharmacy, and suggest a more optimal regimen.

Dietician

A registered dietician or nutritionist evaluates the patient's nutritional status and works with patient, family, and team to determine appropriate nutritional goals.

BARRIERS

Culture Change

➤ Physicians need to adjust from a physician-centered approach to care to one that recognizes the value and importance of an interdisciplinary team.

➤ Midlevel providers who used to have their own panel of patients also need to adjust from being the patient's main provider to being a member of the team.

Change Fatigue

➤ Too much change, too fast, can cause increased staff burnout and turnover.

Cost

➤ Coordination often requires time and effort that may not be obviously billable. Careful attention to reimbursement opportunity is essential. Although payments to midlevel providers are less than those for physicians, the volume, accessibility, and ability to document care coordination of these providers can make these team members cost-effective to a practice (see Chapter 15, Billing Opportunities).

SOLUTIONS

1. Recruit team members with the motivation and skills necessary to manage frail older patients, preferably those having training or experience in geriatrics.

➤ Strong staff support is necessary to coordinate care outside the examination room, such as phone calls, home care agencies, subspecialty care, home equipment, social services, and transition of care.

2. Identify high-risk patients.

➤ Nurses can screen patients for geriatric conditions such as falls, incontinence, and cognitive impairment by using reminders in the electronic medical record.

3. Manage the most complex cases with weekly interdisciplinary team conferences.

4. Utilize shared visits.

➤ In a shared visit with an MD and a midlevel provider, the MD can bill at a higher level and the midlevel provider can do the follow-up and coordination of care.

5. Communicate effectively.

➤ All team members are experts in their field. Respect their opinions and value their perspectives.

➤ Ask specific questions if possible; share your goals for their involvement.

➤ Provide feedback.

> ➤ Identify tools that were particularly helpful, eg, patient education material, electronic business cards.

> ➤ Appreciate innovation and creative solutions to problems, eg, identifying personnel to fill medication boxes.

> ➤ Identify areas for improvement.

➤ Improve team function by providing training based on the work of the Geriatric Interdisciplinary Team Training initiative (www.gittprogram.org).

6. Utilize effective transition of care models.

➤ *Intensive case management by advanced practice nurses (APNs):* Naylor et al[2] demonstrated a decreased rate of readmission and emergency department visits and decreased care cost when elderly patients with congestive heart failure were followed up by an APN after discharge. The APN met with the inpatient team to become familiar with the discharge plan, and then made frequent home visits for patient education and assessment during a 6-week period. After 6 weeks, patients returned to the clinic for further follow-up by their primary care physician. Boling et al[2], using a similar transitional care model, demonstrated cost savings of $1.3 million to health care systems given the prevention of readmission and emergency department visits for frail elders.

➤ *APNs as patient educators and navigators:* Coleman et al[3] focused on patient education and personal health records. In their study, APNs (acting as coaches) provides health education and accompanied recently hospitalized patients to their postdischarge visit to improve communication between the hospital team, primary care provider, and patients/caregiver. Coleman et al also demonstrated reduction in health care utilization.

PATIENT FOLLOW-UP

In the case of Mr E. G., the NP was able to coordinate cardiology follow-up, confirm the medication regimen, and educate the patient about congestive heart failure and the importance of medication compliance. The social worker/case manager assisted in arranging transportation, application to Medicaid for personal care aide support, and transition of the patient back to the ambulatory care setting for further care.

TAKE-HOME POINTS

1. Nonphysician providers deliver key services for older patients, especially in the areas of care coordination and care transitions.

2. Many practice settings benefit from these services, which are reimbursed if appropriately documented.

USEFUL RESOURCES

American Academy of Nurse Practitioners (http://aanp.org/AANPCMS2).

American Academy of Physician Assistants (www.aapa.org).

National Coalition for Care Coordination (N3C). Overview of current initiatives. March 2009 (www.socialworkleadership.org/nsw/news/N3C_Initiative_Overview_Final.pdf).

Mezey M, Boltz M, Esterson J, Mitty E. Evolving models of geriatric nursing care. *Geriatr Nurs.* 2005;26(1):11–15.

Nutting PA. Initial lessons from the first national demonstration project on practice transformation to a patient-centered medical home. *Ann Fam Med.* 2009;7(3):254–260.

Stock RD, Reece D, Cesario L. Developing a comprehensive interdisciplinary senior heathcare practice. *J Am Geriatr Soc.* 2004;52:2128–2133.

REFERENCES

1. Naylor M, Brooten DA, Campbell RL, Maislin G, McCauley KM, Schwartz JS. Transitional care of older adults hospitalized with heart failure: a randomized controlled trial. *J Am Geriatr Soc.* 2004;52(5):675–684.

2. Boling PA, Smigelski CW, et al. Transitional model of care: Bridging inpatient to outpatient care [abstract P518]. *J Am Geriatr Soc.* 2004;52:4(suppl):S194.

3. Coleman E, Parry C, Chalmers S, Min SJ. The care transitions intervention: results of a randomized controlled trial. *Ann Intern Med.* 2006;166(17):1822–1828.

CHAPTER | TWENTY-SIX

Medication Management

Steven M. Handler, MD, MS, CMD

Kevin T. Bain, PharmD, MPH

CASE

You just joined a primary care group practice where the majority of patients are older adults ($\geq$ 65 years) who have multiple comorbidities and are high utilizers of prescription medications. As part of your new position, you have also been asked to see patients in a local nursing home that cares for patients with short- and long-term stays. You are wondering what information you need to know or have access to in order to appropriately prescribe and monitor medications for older adults.

OPPORTUNITIES

➤ Physicians and their patients rely heavily on pharmacotherapy to palliate symptoms, improve functional status and quality of life, cure or manage disease, and prolong survival. Since older adults have multiple comorbidities and are high utilizers of prescription medications, pharmacotherapy represents the most frequently used and misused forms of therapy. Specifically, in the United States, over two-thirds of persons 65 years and older use prescription and over-the-counter drugs; this age group accounts for about one-third of all prescription drug use.[1] Managing the use of medications in older adults is a complex process and requires an understanding of normal changes in pharmacodynamics (how the body responds to a medication) and pharmacokinetics (how the body handles a medication) that occur with aging.

BARRIERS

Significant challenges exist in appropriately prescribing and monitoring medications in older adults. These include:

➤ Obtaining and maintaining a complete medication history, especially during care transitions

➤ Assessing medication adherence and determining which patients may benefit from help with medication management

➤ Determining how to prescribe medications appropriately by understanding:

  ➤ pharmacodynamic and pharmacokinetic changes that occur with aging

  ➤ clinically significant drug-drug and drug-disease interactions

  ➤ potentially inappropriate medications to avoid in older adults

➤ Determining how to monitor medications appropriately by understanding:

  ➤ which medications should be monitored

  ➤ which laboratory parameters should be assessed for the medications that require laboratory monitoring

  ➤ laboratory monitoring intervals for each medication to be monitored

➤ Determining how to discontinue unnecessary medications without causing an adverse drug withdrawal event (a clinically significant set of symptoms or signs caused by the removal of a medication)

➤ Determining whether an adverse drug event (injury resulting from a medical intervention related to a medication) has occurred and, if an event is plausible, possibly reporting it to the Food and Drug Administration (FDA).

SOLUTIONS

➤ *Obtaining and maintaining a complete medication history. Use tools and techniques such as:*

  ➤ Conducting a "brown bag" medication assessment by asking your patients to place all their medications into a brown bag and bring them to their next visit, and then carefully reviewing each medication by using the following form: www.ohiopatientsafety.org/meds/ Brown%20Bag/BBMedicationReviewForm1.doc.

➤ Suggesting that your patients complete and maintain a personal health record containing medical and medication information: www.caretransitions.org/documents/phr.doc.

➤ Detecting changes in medications that may occur during transitional care by using the Medication Discrepancy Tool©: www.caretransitions.org/downloadmdt.asp.

➤ *Assessing and assisting with medication adherence. Use the four-item Morisky scale (Box 26-1).*

➤ *Determining how to prescribe medications appropriately*:

➤ Pharmacodynamic changes that occur with aging (Table 26-1)

➤ As a general rule, the body's response to a medication, particularly its adverse effects, is often enhanced rather than reduced in older adults.

➤ Pharmacokinetic changes that occur with aging, including the absorption, distribution, metabolism, and elimination of medications (Table 26-2)

➤ As a general rule, the most clinically significant pharmacokinetic changes that occur with aging affect the body's metabolism and elimination of medications.

➤ Clinically significant drug-drug and drug-disease interactions:

➤ Refer to the consensus list of drug-drug interactions likely to be encountered in your practice shown in Table 26-3.

➤ Common drug-disease interactions are given at www.merck.com/ mkgr/mmg/tables/6t5.jsp.

➤ See the Cockcroft-Gault equation for estimating creatinine clearance (Box 26-2) and a consensus guideline for primarily renally cleared medications prescribed for older adults (Table 26-4).

➤ Potentially inappropriate medications to avoid in older adults:

➤ See the most recent (2003) Beers criteria at http://archinte.ama-assn.org/cgi/content/full/163/22/2716.

> ### Box 26-1 Morisky Self-reported Measure of Medication Adherence
>
> 1. Do you ever forget to take your medicine?
>
> 2. Are you careless at times about taking your medicine?
>
> 3. When you feel better, do you sometimes stop taking your medicine?
>
> 4. Sometimes if you feel worse when you take your medicine, do you stop taking it?
>
> Source: Morisky DE, Green LW, Levine DM. Concurrent and predictive validity of a self-reported measure of medication adherence. *Med Care*. 1986;24(1):67–74.

➤ *Determining how to monitor medications appropriately. See Table 26-5 for information on which medications should be monitored, which laboratory parameters should be assessed, and laboratory monitoring intervals.*

➤ *Determining how to discontinue unnecessary medications without causing an adverse drug withdrawal event. See Table 26-6 for information on which medications are commonly associated with such events.*

➤ *Detecting and reporting adverse drug events:*

  ➤ It is good practice to place on your differential diagnosis for every geriatric-aged patient the possibility that all new signs, symptoms, and changes in cognitive and/or functional status may be associated with an adverse drug event.

  ➤ Report all new definitive and/or plausible adverse drug events to MedWatch, the FDA Safety Information and Adverse Event Reporting Program: www.fda.gov/downloads/Safety/MedWatch/HowToReport/ DownloadForms/ucm082725.pdf.

➤ *Other strategies to consider:*

  ➤ Collaborate with a pharmacist who specializes in prescribing and monitoring in older adults, medication therapy management, or drug regimen reviews.

  ➤ As covered in other chapters, use an electronic medical record with computerized decision support that includes older adult prescribing and monitoring guidance. See Chapter 18, Medication Refills.

TABLE 26-1 Pharmacodynamic Changes That Occur With Aging

Drug Class	Drug Subclass or Specific Drug	Prescribing Implication	Effect of Aging
Analgesics	NSAIDs	Acute and chronic gastrointestinal mucosal damage	↑
	Opioid analgesics	Analgesic effect, constipation, sedation	↑ ↑
Anticoagulants	Warfarin	Prothrombin time, bleeding risk	↑
Antihypertensives	Calcium-channel blockers	Antihypertensive effect	↑
Benzodiazepines	Especially long-acting agents (eg, diazepam, flurazepam)	Dizziness, memory impairment, sedation	↑ ↑
β-Adrenergic antagonists	Labetalol	Bradycardic response	↓

Sources: Cook PJ, Flanagan R, James IM. *Br Med J (Clin Res Ed)*. Diazepam tolerance: effect of age, regular sedation, and alcohol. 1984;289(6441):351–353.

Platten HP, Schweizer E, Dilger K, Mikus G, Klotz U. Pharmacokinetics and the pharmacodynamic action of midazolam in young and elderly patients undergoing tooth extraction. *Clin Pharmacol Ther*. 1998;63(5):552–560.

Bowie MW, Slattum PW. Pharmacodynamics in older adults: a review. *Am J Geriatr Pharmacother*. 2007;5(3):263–303.

Scott JC, Stanski DR. Decreased fentanyl and alfentanil dose requirements with age: a simultaneous pharmacokinetic and pharmacodynamic evaluation. *J Pharmacol Exp Ther*. 1987;240(1):159–166.

Shepherd AM, Hewick DS, Moreland TA, Stevenson IH. Decreased fentanyl and alfentanil dose requirements with age. A simultaneous pharmacokinetic and pharmacodynamic evaluation. *Br J Clin Pharmacol*. 1977;4(3):315–320.

Bressler R, Bahl JJ. Principles of drug therapy for the elderly patient. *Mayo Clin Proc*. 2003;78(12):1564–1577.

Abernethy DR, Schwartz JB, Plachetka JR, Todd EL, Egan JM. Comparison in young and elderly patients of pharmacodynamics and disposition of labetalol in systemic hypertension. *Am J Cardiol*. 1987;60(8):697–702.

TABLE 26-2 Pharmacokinetic Changes That Occur With Aging

Parameter	Effect of Aging	Effect of Disease/Factor	Prescribing Implications
Absorption (oral)	Rate and extent are usually unaffected	Achlorhydria, concurrent drug therapy, tube feedings	Drug-drug and drug-food interactions are more likely than the normal aging process to alter absorption
Absorption (transdermal)	Rate and extent are usually unaffected	Transdermal absorption may be reduced because of diminished blood flow to the skin; in others, it may be enhanced because aging skin atrophies and becomes thinner	Since there is conflicting information on transdermal absorption, consider that lower doses may be therapeutic
Absorption (intramuscular and subcutaneous)	Rate and extent are usually reduced	Aging decreases muscle mass, and blood perfusion to the muscle and subcutaneous tissues is diminished from diseases commonly affecting older adults such as cardiovascular disease	Lower doses may be therapeutic
Distribution	Increased fat:water ratio; decreased plasma protein, particularly albumin	CHF, ascites, and other conditions will increase body water	Fat-soluble drugs (eg, diazepam, valproic acid) have a larger volume of distribution and often prolonged elimination half-lives; highly protein-bound drugs (eg, phenytoin, warfarin) have a greater (active) free concentration
Metabolism	Decreased liver mass and liver blood flow may decrease drug metabolism	Smoking, genotype, concurrent drug therapy, and alcohol and caffeine intake may have a greater effect than the normal aging process	Lower doses may be therapeutic; see Table 26-3 on drug-drug interactions
Elimination	Decreased GFR reduces renal elimination of drugs	Kidney impairment with acute and chronic diseases; decreased muscle mass results in less creatinine production	Serum creatinine is not a reliable measure of kidney function; best to estimate CrCl with the Cockcroft-Gault equation (Box 26-2).

Sources: Delafuente JC. Pharmacokinetic and pharmacodynamic alterations in the geriatric patient. *Consult Pharm*. 2008;23(4):324–334.

Vasko MR, Cartwright DB, Knochel JP, Nixon JV, Brater DC. Furosemide absorption altered in decompensated congestive heart failure. *Ann Intern Med*. 1985;102(3):314–318.

Solassol I, Caumette L, Bressolle F, et al. Inter- and intra-individual variability in transdermal fentanyl absorption in cancer pain patients. *Oncol Rep*. 2005;14(4):1029–1036.

Holdsworth MT, Forman WB, Killilea TA, et al. Transdermal fentanyl disposition in elderly subjects. *Gerontology*. 1994;40(1):32–37.

Abbreviations: CHF, congestive heart failure; CrCl, creatinine clearance; GFR, glomerular filtration rate.

TABLE 26-3 Consensus List of Clinically Significant and Commonly Encountered Drug-Drug Interactions

Drug Class or Specific Drug	Precipitant Drug Class or Drug
Anticoagulants (anisindione, dicumarol, warfarin)	Thyroid hormones (levothyroxine, liothyronine, liotrix, thyroid, dextrothyroxine)
Benzodiazepines (alprazolam, triazolam)	Azole antifungal agents (fluconazole, itraconazole, ketoconazole)
Carbamazepine	Propoxyphene
Cyclosporine	Rifamycins (rifampin, rifabutin, rifapentine)
Dextromethorphan	MAO inhibitors (isocarboxazid, phenelzine, selegiline, tranylcypromine)
Digoxin	Clarithromycin
Ergot alkaloids (dihydroergotamine, ergotamine, methylsergide)	Macrolide antibiotics (clarithromycin, dirithromycin, erythromycin, troleandomycin)
Estrogen-progestin products (oral contraceptives)	Rifampin
Ganciclovir	Zidovudine
MAO inhibitors (isocarboxazid, phenelzine, selegiline, tranylcypromine)	Anorexiants (amphetamine, benzphetamine, dexfenfluramine, dextroamphetamine, diethylpropion, fenfluramine, mazindol, methamphetamine, phendimetrazine, phentermine, phenylpropanolamine, sibutramine)
MAO inhibitors (isocarboxazid, phenelzine, selegiline, tranylcypromine)	Sympathomimetics (dopamine, ephedrine, isometheptene mucate, mephentermine, metaraminol, phenylephrine, pseudoephedrine)
Meperidine	MAO inhibitors (isocarboxazid, phenelzine, selegiline, tranylcypromine)
Methotrexate	Trimethoprim (trimethoprim-sulfamethoxazole, trimethoprim)
Nitrates (nitroglycerin, isosorbide dinitrate/ mononitrate)	Sildenafil
Pimozide	Macrolide antibiotics (clarithromycin, dirithromycin, erythromycin, troleandomycin)
Pimozide	Azole antifungal agents (fluconazole, itraconazole, ketoconazole)

SSRIs (citalopram, fluoxetine, fluvoxamine, nefazodone, paroxetine, sertraline, venlafaxine)	MAO inhibitors (isocarboxazid, phenelzine, selegiline, tranylcypromine)
Theophyllines	Quinolones (ciprofloxacin, enoxacin)
Theophyllines	Fluvoxamine
Thiopurines (azathioprine, mercaptopurine)	Allopurinol
Warfarin	Sulfinpyrazone
Warfarin	Nonsteroidal anti-inflammatory drugs (celecoxib, diclofenac, etodolac, flurbiprofen, fenoprofen, ibuprofen, indomethacin, ketoprofen, ketorolac, meclofenamate, mefenamic acid, nabumetone, naproxen, oxaprozin, piroxicam, rofecoxib, sulindac, tolmetin)
Warfarin	Cimetidine
Warfarin	Fibric acid derivatives (clofibrate, fenofibrate, gemfibrozil)
Warfarin	Barbiturates (amobarbital, butabarbital, butalbital, mephobarbital, phenobarbital, secobarbital)

Source: Malone DC, Abarca J, Hansten PD, et al. Identification of serious drug-drug interactions: results of the partnership to prevent drug-drug interactions. *J Am Pharm Assoc (2003)*. 2004;44(2):142–151.

Abbreviations: MAO, monoamine oxidase; SSRIs, selective serotonin reuptake inhibitors.

Box 26-2 Estimating Creatinine Clearance (CrCl) by the Cockcroft-Gault Equation

CrCl = [(140 − age)(IBW)/(72 × serum creatinine)] × 0.85 for females,

where age is in years, ideal body weight (IBW) is in kilograms, and serum creatinine is in milligrams per deciliter.

TABLE 26-4 Consensus Guidelines for Primarily Renally Cleared Medications Prescribed for Older Adults

Medication	CrCl (mL/min)	Maximum Suggested Dosage
Acyclovir (for zoster)	10–29	800 mg every 8 hours
	<10	800 mg every 12 hours
Amantadine	30–59	100 mg daily
	15–29	100 mg every other day
	<15	100 mg every 7 days
Chlorpropamide	<50	Avoid use
Ciprofloxacin	<30	500 mg daily
Colchicine	<10	Avoid use
Cotrimoxazole	15–29	800/160 mg daily
	<15	Avoid use
Gabapentin (for pain)	30–59	600 mg every 12 hours
	15–29	300 every 12 hours
	<15	300 mg daily
Glyburide	<30	Avoid use
Memantine	<30	5 mg every 12 hours
Meperidine	<50	Avoid use
Nitrofurantoin	<60	Avoid use
Probenecid	<50	Avoid use
Propoxyphene	<10	Avoid use
Ranitidine	<50	150 mg daily
Rimantadine	<50	100 mg daily
Spironolactone	<30	Avoid use
Triamterene	<30	Avoid use
Valacyclovir (for zoster)	30–49	1000 mg twice daily
	10–29	1000 mg daily
	<10	500 mg daily

Source: Hanlon JT, Aspinall SL, Semla TP, et al. Consensus guidelines for oral dosing of primarily renally cleared medications in older adults. *J Am Geriatr Soc*. 2009;57(2):335–340.

Abbreviation: CrCl, creatinine clearance.

TABLE 26-5 Laboratory Monitoring Parameters and Intervals for Clinically Important Medications Prescribed for Older Adults

Medication Class or Specific Medication	Laboratory Monitoring Parameter	Suggested Interval (months)
Angiotensin II receptor blockers (eg, losartan, valsartan)	Serum potassium level	6
Angiotensin-converting enzyme inhibitors (eg, captopril, enalapril, lisinopril)	Serum potassium level	6
Amiodarone	Serum liver function tests	6
Amiodarone	Thyroid-stimulating hormone level	6
Antidiabetic medications (eg, metformin, glyburide, insulin)	Fasting serum glucose or glycated hemoglobin level	6
Antipsychotic medications (eg, haloperidol, risperidone, quetiapine)	Fasting serum glucose or glycated hemoglobin level	6
Antipsychotic medications (eg, haloperidol, risperidone, quetiapine)	Serum lipid panel	6
Carbamazepine	Trough serum carbamazepine level	6
Cyclosporine	Trough serum cyclosporine level	3
Digoxin	Serum blood urea nitrogen and serum creatinine level	6
Digoxin	Trough serum digoxin level	6
Diuretics (eg, furosemide, hydrochlorothiazide, spironolactone)	Serum sodium and potassium level	3
Erythropoiesis-stimulating agents (eg, epoetin alfa, darbepoetin alfa)	Complete blood count	1
Fibrates (eg, fenofibrate, clofibrate)	Complete blood count	6
Fibrates (eg, fenofibrate, clofibrate)	Serum liver function tests	6
Glucocorticoids, oral	Fasting serum glucose or glycated hemoglobin level	3

(continued)

TABLE 26-5 *(continued)*

Medication Class or Specific Medication	Laboratory Monitoring Parameter	Suggested Interval (months)
Lithium	Trough serum lithium level	3
Metformin	Serum blood urea nitrogen and creatinine level	6
Niacin	Fasting serum glucose or glycated hemoglobin level	6
Niacin	Serum liver function tests	6
Phenobarbital	Trough serum phenobarbital level	6
Phenytoin	Trough serum phenytoin level	3
Primidone	Trough serum primidone level	6
Procainamide	Trough serum procainamide or *N*-acetyl-procainamide level	6
Quinidine	Trough serum quinidine level	6
Salicylate (eg, aspirin. >1200 mg/day, salsalate, choline magnesium trisalicylate)	Trough serum salicylate level	6
Statins (eg, lovastatin, simvastatin)	Serum liver function tests	6
Theophylline	Trough serum theophylline level	3
Thyroid medications (eg, levothyroxine, triiodothyronine, propylthiouracil)	Thyroid-stimulating hormone level	6
Ticlopidine	Complete blood count with neutrophil count	3
Tricyclic antidepressants (eg, amitriptyline, desipramine, imipramine)	Trough serum tricyclic antidepressant level	12
Valproic acid	Trough serum valproic acid level	3
Warfarin	International normalization ratio	1

Source: Handler SM, Shirts BH, Perera S, Becich MJ, Castle NG, Hanlon JT. Frequency of laboratory monitoring of chronic medications administered to nursing facility residents: results of a national Internet-based study. *Consult Pharm*. 2008;23(5):387–395.

TABLE 26-6 Medications Commonly Associated With Adverse Drug Withdrawal Events

Medication Class or Specific Medication	Type of Withdrawal Reaction	Withdrawal Event
α-Antagonist antihypertensives	P	Agitation, headache, hypertension, palpitations
Angiotensin-converting enzyme inhibitors	P, D	Heart failure, hypertension
Antianginals	D	Angina (myocardial ischemia)
Anticonvulsants	P, D	Anxiety, depression, seizures
Antidepressants	P, D	Akathisia, anxiety, chills, coryza, gastrointestinal distress, headache, insomnia, irritability, malaise, myalgia, recurrence of depression
Antiparkinson agents	P, D, N	Hypotension, psychosis, pulmonary embolism, rigidity, tremor
Antipsychotics	P	Dyskinesias, insomnia, nausea, restlessness
Baclofen	P, N	Agitation, anxiety, confusion, depression, hallucinations, hypertonia, insomnia, mania, nightmares, paranoia, seizures
Benzodiazepines	P	Agitation, anxiety, confusion, delirium, insomnia, seizures
β-Blockers	P, D	Angina, anxiety, hypertension, myocardial infarction, tachycardia
Corticosteroids	P, N	Anorexia, hypotension, nausea, weakness
Digoxin	D	Heart failure, palpitations
Diuretics	D	Heart failure, hypertension
Histamine-2 blockers	D	Recurrence of esophagitis and indigestion symptoms
Narcotic analgesics	P	Abdominal cramping, anger, anxiety, chills, diaphoresis, diarrhea, insomnia, restlessness
Nonsteroidal anti-inflammatory drugs	D	Recurrence of arthritis and gout symptoms
Sedative/hypnotics (eg, barbiturates)	P	Anxiety, dizziness, muscle twitches, tremor

(continued)

TABLE 26-6 (continued)

Medication Class or Specific Medication	Type of Withdrawal Reaction	Withdrawal Event
Statins	D, N	Cardiogenic shock, early neurologic deterioration, heart failure, myocardial infarction, ventricular arrhythmia

Bain KT, Holmes HM, Beers MH, Maio V, Handler SM, Pauker SG. Discontinuing medications: a novel approach for revising the prescribing stage of the medication-use process. *J Am Geriatr Soc.* 2008;56(10):1946–1952.

Abbreviations: D, exacerbation of underlying condition; N, new set of symptoms; P, physiologic withdrawal.

TAKE-HOME POINTS

➤ Pharmacotherapy represents the most frequently used and misused forms of therapy in older adults.

➤ Managing the use of medications in older adults is a complex process and requires an understanding of normal pharmacodynamic and pharmacokinetic changes that occur with aging.

➤ Have readily available a number of resources that can improve appropriate prescribing and monitoring of older adults to reduce the likelihood of adverse drug events.

USEFUL RESOURCES

Geriatrics at Your Fingertips (www.geriatricsatyourfingertips.org/).

Drug-drug interaction look-up (http://medicine.iupui.edu/clinpharm/DDIs/table.asp).

Merck Manual of Clinical Geriatrics (Chapter 6, Clinical Pharmacology). at (www.merck.com/mkgr/mmg/sec1/ch6/ch6a.jsp).

Quality indicators for appropriate medication use in vulnerable elders. Assessing Care of Vulnerable Elders (ACOVE) Project (www.rand.org/pubs/reprints/2005/RP1134.pdf).

American Society of Consultant Pharmacists (www.ascp.com/).

American Geriatrics Society (www.americangeriatrics.org/).

American Medical Directors Association (www.amda.com).

REFERENCE

1. Qato DM, Alexander GC, Johnson M, Schumm P, Lindau, ST. Use of prescription and over-the-counter medications and dietary supplements among older adults in the United States. JAMA. 2008 Dec 24;300(24):2867–78.

CHAPTER TWENTY-SEVEN

The Electronic Medical Record (EMR): Considerations for Geriatric Care

Audrey Chun, MD

THE MULTISPECIALTY PRACTICE EXPERIENCE WITH EMR PLANNING

Your medical director has decided to implement an electronic medical record (EMR) for your multispecialty practice. You've been asked to serve on the planning committee to choose a system and help design templates that are generic enough for use by all providers in the practice. As a physician in a primary care group that cares for a large number of older adults and patients with multiple morbidities, you wonder how implementing this new system will affect your efficiency and personalized care of patients. You also wonder how an EMR might enhance the care you give to your patients.

OPPORTUNITIES

Electronic medical records (also known as electronic health records, or EHRs) have been both vilified and glorified in relation to patient care. While not required, an EMR can facilitate many aspects of care coordination, practice improvement, and communications. Additionally, when selected and used properly, EMRs can have distinct advantages for practices caring for older adults.

➤ *Improved screening:* Screening reminders can be embedded for geriatric-specific conditions such as incontinence, memory loss, and falls as well as routine health maintenance.

➤ *Improved care coordination:*

1. Through registries and alerts (panel management tools), identification of at-risk patients or those requiring specific tests/screens can improve adherence to guidelines for diseases and health maintenance.

2. Early identification of patients admitted to the emergency department or hospital enhances information exchange and transitions of care.

3. Additionally, EMR use facilitates communications between providers and assists with medication reconciliation, messaging, and prescription faxing.

➤ *Improved efficiency:* Automatic charge entry, documentation templates, patient care reminders, abnormal test flags, and flowsheets can increase time with patients by decreasing paperwork and time spent on information gathering for patient visits.

➤ *Improved patient satisfaction:* Patients may feel empowered through interactive Web sites with 24-hour access that can help schedule appointments, ease communication with their physicians, and/or facilitate finding results.

➤ *Improved patient safety:* The incidence of medical errors can be decreased through alerts for drug-drug interactions, duplicate medications, and potentially inappropriate dosing.

➤ *Increased revenues:* Increased financial incentives from insurers for EMR implementation along with automatic charge submission can increase practice revenues over time.

➤ *Improved physician satisfaction:* Physician satisfaction may increase because of the perception of improved quality of care.[1,2]

CHALLENGES

Despite these advantages, there are real challenges that hinder the successful implementation of an EMR.

➤ *Cost:* Initial start-up costs, both direct and related to time for research, planning, and implementation, without assured cost savings in the future, are a major barrier to considering EMR implementation.

➤ *Compatibility:* The EMR must be compatible with other systems to enable access to hospital laboratory results, messaging other practices, retrieval of reports, and for search functions.

➤ *Input of records:* Outside paper-based records must be scanned or input to the EMR, and these files are difficult to subsequently search, open, and print.

➤ *Technical support:* Varying technical expertise by users and variable support from EMR vendors affects the ability to successfully implement and maintain a useful system.

➤ *Staff and physician culture change:* Any major practice change requires a willingness to interact with new technology, change workflows, and devote time to planning and implementation.

➤ *Potential inefficiency of care:* There may be an initial decline in efficiency when staff members are learning the system, and if the system is not a good fit, the efficiency may not improve with time.

➤ *Need for customization:* A "cookie-cutter" approach with templates may increase inappropriate screening and tests if they are unable to account for patient wishes or prognosis.

➤ *Unrealistic expectations:* Unmanaged expectations related to the EMR can create dissatisfaction by staff and physicians. In our case, this was especially challenging as many users hoped that the EMR would address problems that were, in fact, more systems-based and not likely to be changed by an EMR.

➤ *Patient dissatisfaction:* There is the potential for more time spent with the technology than with the patient.

SOLUTIONS

1. Prepare.

➤ Create a vision/goal statement of what you hope the EMR will help facilitate in your practice.[3,4]

➤ Identify stakeholders and make sure they have representation in the process. This will improve buy-in for any workflow changes and also help make sure the EMR chosen is the best fit for the practice. The planning committee should include representatives with expertise in nursing, finance, insurance, and compliance issues.

➤ Designate an EMR champion. This person should have influence in the practice to facilitate culture changes.

➤ Prioritize needs and match to functions and support available in the proposed EMR (Table 27-1).

➤ Evaluate current workflow. Determine whether your EMR will mimic your paper flow or whether there will be changes to adapt to the EMR. Radical changes to workflow to accommodate the EMR will likely meet extreme resistance from physicians and staff. However, it is also an opportunity to reconsider office flow and efficiency issues.

➤ Plan your budget. How much can you realistically afford to invest?

➤ Limit EMR selection to those that interface with your current systems.

➤ Prepare requests for proposals.

TABLE 27-1 Checklist for Inquiries of EMR Functionality

Function	Must Have	Nice to Have	Don't Need	Rank
Billing and documentation:				
Coding advisor				
Automated charges				
Order and retrieve results:				
Laboratory tests				
Other studies				
Consultations				
Tracking (flags duplicates, abnormal results, missing results)				
Laboratory tests				
Studies				
Consultations				
Registries				
Notification of emergency department/hospital admission				
Prescription writer				
E-prescribing (connects to pharmacies)				
Drug-drug interaction alert				
Duplicate drug alert				
Drug cost alert				

Drug dosing alert				
Drug-allergy alert				
Health screening reminders				
Secure interactive Web site or external e-mail for patients				
Scheduling				
Reports for QI or research				
Remote access				
Flowsheet capability (vital signs, laboratory studies)				
Interface with internal and external laboratories				
Internal e-mail				
Telephone message documentation				
Patient education				
Scanning				
Electronic faxing (laboratory results, reports, letters, consultations)				
Alerts (health maintenance, follow-up)				
Decision support tools				
Security				
Documentation of patient teach-back with medications/ recommendations				
GERIATRICS-SENSITIVE				
Clear advance care planning documentation areas:				
Code status				
Goals of care				
Health care proxy/agent				

(continued)

TABLE 27-1 *(continued)*

Function	Must Have	Nice to Have	Don't Need	Rank
Flexible contact fields for emergencies or for care communications				
Hospital admission alert				
Supports billing and documentation for prolonged services and coordination of care				
Flowsheets, screening reminders, or decision support for common geriatric conditions:				
Urinary incontinence				
Memory loss				
Falls				
Functional assessments				
Screening alert function allows for documenting if inappropriate based on prognosis or patient wishes				
Patient education				
Font size adjustable				
Medication list prints in easy-to-understand instructions				
Option for connection to online patient handouts or link to office handouts				

2. Choose and purchase.

➤ Estimate cost of the EMR and time to return on investment.

➤ Inquire into the amount of technical support from the vendor, including options for upgrades and changes as your practice changes.

➤ Choose best fits based on priorities.

➤ Visit practices with similar characteristics to yours that are using the systems you are considering.

3. Implement.

➤ Preparation for training and culture changes should begin before implementation (see Chapters 11 and 23 for additional tips on team building and communications) and should include:

> ➤ Plans for reduced scheduling during EMR go-live

> ➤ Time for training users

> ➤ Plans for chart abstraction or time-limited use of paper charts during the transition

> ➤ Workflow changes, as needed and planned

TAKE-HOME POINTS

➤ Careful planning will improve the chances of choosing an EMR with the most successful implementation and overall satisfaction with the system.

➤ Manage expectations of patients, staff, and physicians. The EMR is one tool that can help facilitate good patient care and improve efficiency. It is not a replacement for direct communication and good clinical practices.

USEFUL RESOURCES

American Academy of Family Physicians

➤ Online resource for health information technology, including EHR selection.

➤ (www.centerforhit.org/online/chit/home.html).

American College of Physicians

➤ Roadmap for EHR adoption.

➤ (www.acponline.org/running_practice/technology/ehr/roadmap/).

➤ AmericanEHR Partners is a web-based resource for EHR system selection/implementation developed by the American College of Physicians and Cientis Technologies.

➤ (http://www.americanehr.com).

American Medical Association

➤ Selecting health information technology:

➤ (www.ama-assn.org/ama/pub/physician-resources/solutions-managing-your-practice/health-information-technology/putting-hit-practice/selecting-hit.shtml).

Healthcare Information and Management Systems Society

➤ Comparison of EMRs and other health information technology.

➤ (www.himss.org).

REFERENCES

1. DesRoches CM, Campbell EG, Rao SR, et al. Electronic health records in ambulatory care—a national survey of physicians. *N Engl J Med*. 2008;359(1):50–60.

2. Edsall RL, Adler KG. An EHR user-satisfaction survey: advice from 408 family physicians. *Fam Pract Manag*. 2005;12(9):29–35.

3. Adler KG. How to select an electronic health record system. *Fam Pract Manag*. 2005;12(2):55–62.

4. Lorenzi NM, Kouroubali A, Detmer DE, Bloomrosen M. How to successfully select and implement electronic health records (EHR) in small ambulatory practice settings. *BMC Med Inform Decis Mak*. 2009;9:15.

CHAPTER TWENTY-EIGHT

Improving Care Transitions for Older Adults

Alicia I. Arbaje, MD, MPH

MS MARY VEE'S EXPERIENCE

Ms Mary Vee is an 81-year-old woman with a complex medical history and social situation. She has a total of six chronic conditions, including congestive heart failure (CHF), diabetes, and hypertension. She has four physicians who manage her care, and she is taking nine medications. She lives at home with her husband, who has dementia, and she is his primary caregiver. They have one daughter, who has a family of her own and lives 20 miles away.

Ms Vee has been in the hospital three times during the last 6 months for CHF exacerbations. She has required two rehabilitation stays and three episodes of home care because of debility and medication changes after these hospitalizations. Across all of these health care settings, she has had a total of eight new physicians, 25 nurses, and seven rehabilitation therapists. She has had four new medication lists prepared, and she has been prescribed three new medications. Her primary care provider (PCP) was not aware of Ms Vee's hospitalizations and medication changes until after discharge, when he was called to sign home care orders.

INTRODUCTION

Transitional care refers to a set of actions designed to ensure the coordination and continuity of health care as patients transfer between different locations or different levels of care. Optimal care includes the following elements:

➤ Logistical arrangements related to the care transition

➤ Patient/caregiver education to prepare them for what to expect at the next site of care

➤ Coordination among the health care professionals involved in executing the patient's care plan

OPPORTUNITIES

Care transitions are becoming more common and represent potential "danger points," or moments that leave patients at risk for lapses in their care. Older adults are less able to tolerate these lapses. Optimal transitional care can result in improved outcomes for older adults, including the following:

➤ More effective implementation of care plans because all those involved in the patient's care are aware of the medical history, pending tests, new diagnoses, and changes in medication regimens

➤ Less time spent tracking down information about a patient's hospitalization after the patient has been discharged

➤ Awareness of the patient's admission to the hospital, and improved communication with inpatient and home care providers

➤ Decreased medication errors and adverse events

➤ Decreased emergency department visits and readmission rates

➤ Improved provider, patient, and caregiver satisfaction

CHALLENGES

1. Variation in patient transitional care needs.

➤ Needs depend on illness, social situation, and type of transition.

➤ Patients who live alone, have unmet functional needs, or have limited self-management ability may be at higher risk for early hospital readmission and thus need particular attention during care transitions.

➤ Transitions to home requiring home care are often the most risky, perhaps because patients are not sick enough to qualify for a skilled nursing facility stay, but they are not well enough to go home without assistance.

2. Lack of provider education and feedback.

➤ Providers often are not trained to execute effective care transitions, including preparing timely and effective discharge summaries.

➤ Providers often have not practiced in settings where they transfer patients.

➤ Providers are often not aware of whether the patient experiences an optimal transition or whether the receiving provider at the next site of care has sufficient information to continue to execute the care plan.

3. Difficulty accessing colleagues.

➤ Inpatient and outpatient providers may not have the time or resources to overcome the difficulties in accessing colleagues at the previous or next site of care.

➤ Providers may lack the knowledge of who is the responsible provider or how to reach him or her.

➤ Busy schedules may not allow for an appropriate time to talk about the patient's care plan.

4. Lack of resources.

➤ Transitional care activities that involve care coordination are largely not billable in the current reimbursement system.

SOLUTIONS

1. Set expectations.

Overall

➤ Shift from the concept of "discharge" to "transfer with continuous management."

➤ Begin transfer planning upon or before admission.

➤ Incorporate patient's/caregivers' preferences into plan.

➤ Identify a patient's social support and function (how will this patient care for herself after transfer?).

➤ Collaborate with practitioners across settings to formulate and execute a common care plan.

For the sending team

➤ Ensure that the patient is stable for transfer.

➤ Make sure the patient and/or caregiver understands the purpose of the transfer.

➤ Check that the patient/caregiver understands his or her coverage.

➤ Confirm that the receiving institution is capable and prepared.

➤ Transmit the care plan, orders, and clinical summary before the patient's arrival.

➤ Be sure the patient has a timely follow-up appointment.

For the receiving team

➤ Review transfer forms, clinical summary, and orders prior to or upon the patient's arrival.

➤ Incorporate the patient's/caregiver's goals and preferences into the care plan.

➤ Clarify discrepancies regarding the care plan, patient's status, or patient's medications.

2. Tailor communication strategies:

Use different types of communication depending on the situation.

➤ Written (faxes, letters)

➤ Discharge summaries

➤ Consultant recommendation

➤ Electronic (e-mail, text pages)

➤ Notification of admission or start of service

➤ Nonurgent issues

➤ Verbal (telephone, in-person)

➤ Situations of urgency or uncertainty, or when something goes wrong

➤ New diagnoses of cancer or other serious illnesses

➤ Difficult social situations, complicated family dynamics, nuances

3. Follow outcome measures.

Choose one or two to focus on, then expand further once goals are achieved.

For hospital and health systems

➤ Notification of PCP on patient admission

➤ Communication with PCP before discharge

➤ Medication reconciliation at each transfer

➤ Patient satisfaction with preparation for discharge

➤ Safe arrival of patient at destination

➤ Discharge summaries that meet standard quality measures

➤ Timely arrival of discharge summaries

➤ PCP satisfaction with quality of communication

➤ Searchable medical records with easy access

➤ Patient adherence to plan of care at 1 week

➤ Patient show rate to follow-up PCP appointment

For outpatient practices

➤ Provision of records on transfer to hospital

➤ Easy access to provider for communication

➤ Searchable medical records with easy access

➤ Up-to-date medical records

➤ Timely signature of home health care orders

➤ Timely arrival of consultation notes

➤ Regional exchange of health information

For discharge summaries, inclusion of the following elements

➤ Judgment and decision making

➤ Follow-up instructions

➤ New diagnoses

➤ Results of major tests and consultations

➤ Current medication list, specifying changes

➤ Baseline and current functional and cognitive status

TAKE-HOME POINTS

➤ Transitional care is an important element for safe and effective health care.

➤ Poor transitional care is especially dangerous for older adults.

➤ Effective solutions to improve transitional care require a team-based approach.

➤ The following elements are important for ensuring optimal transitional care for older adults:

  ➤ Communication during admission and discharge

  ➤ Timely and quality discharge summaries

  ➤ Medication reconciliation

  ➤ Use of home health care when appropriate

  ➤ Patient/caregiver preparation for next site of care

  ➤ Follow-up telephone call to patient after discharge, ideally within 48 hours

USEFUL RESOURCES

National Transitions of Care Coalition

➤ (www.ntocc.org).

➤ Taking Care of MY Health Care.

➤ MY Medicine List.

Care Transitions Program

➤ (www.caretransitions.org).

➤ Care Transitions Measure (three- or 15-item survey).

➤ Medication Discrepancy Tool.

Society of Hospital Medicine

➤ (www.hospitalmedicine.org).

➤ Quality Improvement Resource Room: BOOSTing Transitions.

CHAPTER TWENTY-NINE

Role of the Family Caregiver

Elizabeth G. Fine, LCSW

Dante Tipiani, MSW

Eileen H. Callahan, MD

MARTHA'S EXPERIENCE

Martha is a 72-year-old Puerto Rican bilingual married woman with a medical history of diabetes and hypertension. She is a retired schoolteacher who has two children from her first marriage and now lives with her second husband, to whom she has been married for the last 15 years. She came to see you at the insistence of her husband, who is concerned about her change in functioning.

Martha's husband accompanied her to the appointment. The patient reported some short-term memory problems. Her husband described a 1-year history of increasing forgetfulness, difficulty remembering appointments and paying her bills; and increased problems managing her medications.

After a dementia workup was completed, Martha and her husband returned to discuss her diagnosis of dementia due to early-stage Alzheimer's disease. Martha did not agree with the diagnosis (a common occurrence in early-stage dementia), but her husband wanted information about what to do next. Where could he learn more about Alzheimer's disease? How should they prepare for the future? What medications were available and where could they locate clinical trials opportunities?

OPPORTUNITIES

In a recent national survey, 65.7 million people reported they are providing care for a chronically ill, disabled, or aged family member or friend during any given year.[1] Martha is in the early stages of dementia, a chronic progressive disorder. She has a family caregiver, her husband. Now is the time for them to learn about the diagnosis and options for treatment and long-term care, discuss the options, and make plans for the future burden of the disease that they will likely encounter.

Advance Directives

Discuss advance directives while Martha is in the early stages of dementia and has the capacity to do so. This discussion should be ongoing as her condition changes.[2] At the time of diagnosis, the following topics should be discussed:

➤ Goals of medical care, as well as long-term care and end-of-life care preferences

➤ Assignment of a health care proxy, completion of a living will, and assignment of a durable power of attorney for legal and financial matters

➤ Present and future financial planning needs, possibly including consultation with an elder-law attorney

Treatment Options

Discuss with Martha and her husband the different treatment options, both nonpharmacologic and pharmacologic. Keep in mind the following issues:

➤ Capacity to make decisions[2] (informed consent)

➤ Cultural preferences (ask about preferences; if language interpretation services are needed, use a trained professional or volunteer interpreter, not a family member or a friend)

➤ Options for palliative (comfort) care and end-of-life hospice care

➤ Referrals (private and public supportive services, geriatric psychiatry, social work, medications, clinical trials)

Safety Issues

Physicians play an important role in education and recommendations about interventions to improve patient safety. Patient diagnosis, stage of disease, and social and financial factors must be considered. These factors need to be carefully evaluated and reevaluated as the disease progresses. Concerns include:

➤ For patients with cognitive impairments, appropriate supervision in the home or another facility

➤ Devices to facilitate safety (eg, Alzheimer's Association Safe Return Program)

➤ Driving safety

➤ Vulnerability to abuse by others and self-neglect

➤ Environmental safety in the home (eg, burn prevention, falls prevention)

➤ Ability to safely manage and take medications

Caregiver Needs

Caregivers require both support and education to optimize care for a person with dementia or other chronic illnesses.

Support: Caregivers often suffer from enormous stress and even depression. Most try to manage their caregiving responsibilities alone. Caregivers should be provided emotional support and education that will help them care for their loved ones at home as long as possible. This is what most caregivers want to do. It is essential that you ask the caregiver one simple question: "How are you doing?"

Education: Providing both the patient and the caregiver with education about the disease with which the patient has been diagnosed will empower them to manage the illness and to prepare for the future. In most cases the physician may not have the time or expertise to provide in-depth education. However, if outpatient team members (eg, social workers, nurse practitioners) are available, they may provide both education and support. Physicians should provide referrals to caregiving organizations—both diagnosis-specific and general. Organizations that provide caregiver support and education are listed in the Useful Resources section at the end of this chapter.

CHALLENGES

Advance Directives

Care can become difficult to coordinate if a patient has not assigned a health care agent. Patients with more advanced dementia or other medical/psychiatric illnesses may not be able to direct their medical care. The following barriers influence preferences regarding care:

➤ Decision-making capacity[2]

➤ Cultural aspects of care (understanding cultural background)

➤ Family dynamics (family members disagreeing with each other; family members unable to take on caregiving roles desired by patient or other family members)

➤ Language barrier

Treatment Options

Every patient and family brings its norms and values for care to the physician's office. Think about the case of Martha and barriers that can develop:

➤ Inability to remember to take prescribed medications

➤ Inability to afford the medication

➤ Denial of the diagnosis on the part of the patient or family

➤ Refusal of a pharmacologic approach

➤ Stigma attached to mental illnesses

Safety Issues

Safety is the most important aspect of patient care. Assess and reassess the following barriers with your patient and caregiver:

➤ No family or family that is unavailable or unreliable

➤ History of getting lost or wandering

➤ History of alcohol or drug abuse

➤ History of depression, suicide attempts

➤ Refusal to stop driving (Also see Chapter 17). Some states have mandatory reporting of unsafe drivers related to some illnesses, but not to others. Other states have permissive reporting, and yet others have no regulations at all. This is a developing field of law, one that does not have a single, uniform, federal rule.[3] There are also ethical and policy questions raised when physician-patient confidentiality (to protect the patient and public) must be balanced against the unintended consequence that reporting may discourage elderly patients from seeking medical care.

➤ Refusal to accept supervision (loss of independence)

➤ Refusal of medications (memory loss, fear of side effects, financial problems)

Elder abuse: Dementia patients are at an increased risk of abuse. Abuse can take different forms:

➤ Financial (bank, Social Security and Medicare/Medicaid fraud, stealing cash or belongings)

➤ Physical (from withholding medications, personal care, and nutrition, to outright assault)

➤ Sexual (indications of sexual abuse include bruising on inner thighs, genital or anal bleeding, and new sexually transmitted diseases)

➤ Emotional/psychological (eg, abusive or belittling language, threats of abandonment, misuse of elder's property [such as using home/yard for drug transactions])

➤ Older adults are vulnerable to all of these forms of abuse by institutional or family/nonfamily in-home caregivers (eg, home health aides)

Caregiver Needs

Family caregivers like Martha's husband frequently neglect their own health care needs, leading to chronic stress, burnout, and illness. In a geriatric practice, clinicians can fail to identify a stressed caregiver. Assess caregiver needs for support and education:

Support

➤ Emotional (anxiety, depression, anger, grief, guilt, etc)

➤ Physical health (lack of medical care, poor diet, lack of exercise)

➤ Spiritual beliefs (loss of faith)

➤ Social isolation (weakened support systems due to friend and family illness/death; neglected friendships)

➤ Family dynamics (eg, lack of family involvement; destructive involvement by family members)

Education

➤ Caregivers who are uneducated about the diagnosis lack the knowledge and/or skills that they will need to help plan for, care for, and manage the patient. For example, patients with dementia, like Martha, can develop other disturbances such as sleep problems, agitation, and hallucinations.[4] Patients with other diseases such as cancer can develop symptoms from the disease or their treatment such as vomiting, pain, fatigue, and delirium.[5]

SOLUTIONS

Health care professionals should be aware of the patient's and caregiver's cultural background and the language in which they choose to communicate. If their language differs from that of the professional, use a professional translation service, either in-person or telephone-based. Do not use the caregiver, family member, or paid companion to translate.

Advance Directives

What kind of medical care would Martha want as her dementia progresses? Contact a palliative care specialist or a geriatrician, who can assist you with this process, if needed. Consultation with a psychiatrist may be indicated to address capacity issues for certain patients. Refer Martha and her husband to a social worker if emotional support and guidance on the implications of advance directives is needed.

The following are important documents to complete:

➤ Living will

➤ Health care proxy, also known as a health care power of attorney (medical decision making). Forms vary by state; complete forms in the state in which the patient resides.

➤ Durable power of attorney. Refer Martha and her husband to an attorney specializing in elder law. The cost of caring for a person with dementia can be financially overwhelming for caregivers. An elder-law attorney can help them financially prepare for the care that Martha may need in the future and also complete a durable power of attorney to give her husband legal authority to make financial and legal decisions. The National Academy of Elder Law Attorneys provides names of local attorneys who can help advise them. The Alzheimer's Association offers free legal and financial information for patients and families.

➤ If no one is available or assigned to be a patient's health care proxy or to have power of attorney, a court-appointed guardian is needed.

Treatment Options

➤ *Nonpharmacologic:*

  ➤ Keeping the brain stimulated through memory aerobic classes may hold some benefit.[6]

➤ A support group will provide an opportunity for Martha to share her feelings and engage socially with others in a relatively judgment-free and safe environment.

➤ Encourage regular exercise for physical health and to enhance cognition as well.[7]

➤ Recent literature points out the merits of mental activities such as crossword puzzles, word search games, sudoku, and even some computer games.[8] Continuing-education classes and senior center programs that promote socialization enhance mental activity.

➤ Martha should purchase a daily calendar to strengthen her independence and sense of control.

➤ Keeping old routines and creating new ones can help give Martha a greater sense of control over her life; make sure not to overschedule. Usually scheduling one activity a day is manageable.

➤ Use a pill box to organize medications. This can help decrease confusion and maximize medication compliance.

➤ To help ease the burden of some responsibilities, arrange for direct deposit of monthly checks (Social Security, Registered Retirement Savings Plan, annuity) and direct withdrawal of monthly bills (telephone, electricity, etc).

➤ *Pharmacologic:*

➤ For the treatment of dementia, choices include cholinesterase inhibitors: donepezil, rivastigmine (patch or pills), galantamine, and the *N*-methyl-D-aspartate (NMDA) receptor antagonist memantine.[9]

➤ There are more than 30 National Institutes of Health–funded research centers across the country that accept patients for clinical trials of new medications seeking Food and Drug Administration approval. The medications under review may offer symptomatic improvement for some patients, although there may be risks associated with participation.

Safety

➤ *Safe Return Identification Bracelet*: Recommend that your patients in the middle and later stages of dementing illness purchase a Safe Return identification bracelet.

➤ Supported by the Alzheimer's Association, these ID bracelets or necklaces are worn by individuals with dementia. In the event that they wander, are lost, or are injured and unable to communicate, the bracelet provides a toll-free number. Callers are connected to a service that contacts designated respondents. The service also works closely with local law enforcement personnel and missing persons reporting systems.

➤ The caregiver can also wear a bracelet. In the event that something should happen to the caregiver, the bracelet alerts authorities that there is a person with dementia at home alone.

➤ *Personal Emergency Response System (PERS):* These are in-home devices that connect to a 24-hour call center with the push of a button. The transmitter is typically worn on a neck pendant or wristband, and it sends a signal to a receiver that is connected to the home telephone line.

➤ *Appropriate supervision:*

➤ *Wandering:* As mentioned earlier, the Safe Return bracelet will help to locate someone if he or she gets lost. However, consider putting an alarm on the door and/or an additional lock out of the person's reach.

➤ *Cooking:* Make sure that the stove elements are turned off after use. To prevent accidental burning—particularly for those persons with dementia who live alone or who are in the middle and later stages of the illness—remove stovetop and oven knobs between uses and hide them in an inaccessible place.

➤ *Managing finances:* Individuals with dementia are vulnerable to becoming victims of fraud and financial abuse. Monitoring or supervision of finances is advised. Early in the illness, patients should name a durable power of attorney to take over their financial responsibilities when they are no longer able to perform them themselves.

➤ *Allowing strangers in the home:* Individuals with dementia will experience impaired judgment as the disease progresses. Adequate supervision is needed to ensure that they do not allow strangers into their homes.

➤ *Increased supervision:* As the illness progresses, patients with dementia will require more supervision, which may be provided by a family member and/or paid home or institutional care workers. A community social worker can assist the caregiver in determining eligibility and completing applications for financial resources such as Medicare, Medicaid, and other services.

➤ *Driving:* Ask patients whether they are currently driving (Also see Chapter 17). Assessing a patient's ability to drive can be difficult. If there is doubt, refer patients to an occupational therapist or driver rehabilitation specialist to evaluate their abilities. Engage in an ongoing discussion about patients' driving abilities, while helping them to plan for alternate means of transportation. Caregivers should be part of this dialogue, as often the caregiver is the one who must enforce the decision to stop driving.

➤ There are legal considerations for physicians with impaired-driver patients. A state-by-state patchwork of laws and regulations creates different obligations (and prohibitions). Must the physician report? May the physician report? The answers largely depend on where the physician practices and where the patient lives.[3]

➤ Physicians are urged to consult with their state's Department of Motor Vehicles and/or legal counsel to ascertain local requirements.

➤ *Elder abuse:* If there is concern that a patient is being neglected or abused, the physician should interview and examine the patient alone. In 1992 The American Medical Association proposed that clinicians in all practice settings screen geriatric patients to identify abuse. Physicians should routinely ask about elder abuse in their daily practice.[10] Several different screening tools are available, but all have issues with implementation or reliability.[11] Simple questions can be asked, such as "Do you feel safe at home?" "Who prepares your meals?" "Who handles your checkbook?"[12] If these questions and/or findings on the physical examination raise reasonable suspicion of elder abuse, the physician should pursue more questioning and offer medical, social, and legal interventions to the patient. Each state has different laws regarding the legal obligations and available agencies. Web sites are listed in the Useful Resources section at the end of the chapter.

Caregiver Needs

Always keep brochures and a list of helpful resources in your office, such as:

➤ Information (brochures, pamphlets, books, Web sites)

➤ Referrals (educational and supportive groups, workshops)

➤ Resources (community- and organization-based knowledge)

Support:

➤ Caregivers of patients with dementia should be referred to a network of support groups offered free of charge by the Alzheimer's Association; this will help them learn how to care for patients. Various online organizations also allow caregivers to connect with others. For some caregivers a connection via telephone can also been helpful; inquire about a telephone support group though the Alzheimer's Association. There are a multitude of other support groups across the country for caregivers dealing with individuals with other diseases such as cancer.

➤ For caregivers who need more help or an expert's assessment, or who do not live near the patient, a private geriatric care manager can provide critical expertise. Geriatric care managers are trained professionals, usually social workers or nurses with a specialized focus on aging and elder care. These professionals can be hired to provide services such as supervising or managing paid home care workers, accompanying patients to medical appointments, or arranging for placement in assisted living facilities or nursing homes. These services are usually not covered by health or long-term care insurance policies; fees may range from $300 to $500 for an initial consultation and care plan and $80 to $150 per hour for services thereafter. Despite the cost, these services are critical for some patients and caregivers, whether local or long-distance. For caregivers with limited financial resources, the local chapter of the Alzheimer's Association can guide these long-distance caregivers to appropriate services.

Education: The Alzheimer's Association is one of the most valuable referrals you can give to your patients with dementing illness and their caregivers. The Alzheimer's Association provides the following invaluable information and resources:

➤ Educational materials and lectures on Alzheimer's disease. These are available both on the Internet and as written material. Materials are available in a variety of languages and are all free of charge. Topics covered include the following:

  ➤ What is Alzheimer's disease?

  ➤ Living with Alzheimer's disease

  ➤ Communicating with the person with Alzheimer's disease

  ➤ Making the home safe

  ➤ Dealing with difficult behavior

  ➤ Caring for the caregivers

➤ A 24-hour hotline at (800) 272-3900 that provides information and support to those affected by Alzheimer's disease and other dementing illnesses

➤ Referral to elder-law attorneys

➤ A list of medical research centers throughout the country that are involved in Alzheimer-related clinical trials

➤ Lists of support groups for individuals with early-stage Alzheimer's disease

➤ Lists of support groups for caregivers

➤ Referrals to home health care agencies

➤ Referrals to programs like adult day care services in the community

➤ Lists of assisted living facilities or skilled nursing facilities

Communication between health care professional and caregivers: Unlike Martha, many patients do not have a caregiver who lives close to them. In addition, many caregivers are not available to attend appointments with the patient; rather, a paid companion may come with the patient. Reaching out to the primary caregiver is essential to ensure optimal care and avoid miscommunication. The physician should establish guidelines for communication early on. This can be accomplished via telephone, e-mail, or written correspondence (with written letters faxed or sent home with the home companion) with the patient's primary caregiver.

While this chapter focuses on the role of the family caregiver in Alzheimer's disease, it serves as a framework for dealing with other dementias, chronic illnesses, and disabilities. Other disease-specific Web sites exist for caregivers and are listed at the end of the chapter.

TAKE-HOME POINTS

- Providing Martha and her husband with a diagnosis of Alzheimer's disease is only the beginning of a long and complicated journey with this couple.

- Ask Martha's husband early on how he is coping. If the caregiver is coping well, he will be better able to care for the patient.

- Help connect caregivers with valuable resources as early as possible regarding the following topics, as appropriate:

  - Advance directives

  - Legal and financial planning

  - Information and education about the diagnosis

  - Support groups for patients and caregivers

  - Individual and family therapists

  - Home care services, assisted living facilities, and nursing homes

- Be sensitive to and aware of the cultural and linguistic aspects of providing care to a multicultural population. Use professional translation services, either in-person or telephone-based.

- Continuously monitor for abuse and neglect of your elderly patients; those with dementia are most vulnerable.

USEFUL RESOURCES

➤ Alzheimer's Association (www.alz.org).

➤ Alzheimer's Research Foundation (www.alzinfo.org).

➤ American Geriatrics Society (www.americangeriatrics.org).

➤ National Association of Professional Geriatric Care Managers (www.caremanager.org).

➤ National Academy of Elder Law Attorneys (www.naela.org).

➤ National Institutes of Health–Funded Clinical Research Centers (www.nia.nih.gov/Alzheimers).

➤ Family Caregiver Support Network (www.caregiversupportnetwork.org).

➤ Family Caregiver Alliance–National Center on Caregiving (www.caregiver.org/caregiver/jsp/home.jsp).

➤ National Family Caregivers Association (www.thefamilycaregiver.org).

➤ National Family Caregiver Support Program (www.agingcarefl.org/services/programs/NationalSupport).

➤ Caring Connections (www.caringinfo.org).

➤ The Fisher Center for Alzheimer's Research Foundation Community (www.alzinfo.org/community).

➤ Today's Caregiver (www.caregiver.com).

➤ Division of Motor Vehicles (www.dmv.com).

➤ American Cancer Society (www.cancer.org).

➤ Cancer Care (www.cancercare.org).

➤ American Bar Association Commission on Law and Aging (www.abanet.org/aging/).

➤ National Center on Elder Abuse (www.ncea.aoa.gov).

➤ Long-term Care Ombudsman Resource Center (www.ltcombudsman.org).

➤ Administration on Aging (www.aoa.gov).

➤ Medic Alert Foundation (www.medicalert.org).

➤ American Medical Association Caregiver Health Web site (http://www.ama-assn.org/ama/pub/physician-resources/public-health/promoting-healthy-lifestyles/geriatric-health/caregiver-health.shtml)

➤ American Medical Association in cooperation with the National Highway Traffic Safety Administration. *Physician's Guide to Assessing and Counseling Older Drivers*. 2010 (www.ama-assn.org/go/olderdrivers).

REFERENCES

1. Executive Summary of the National Alliance for Caregiving, in collaboration with AARP and funded by the MetLife Foundation on Caregiving in the United States. Available at: www.caregiving.org. Accessed February 9, 2010.

2. Appelbaum PS. Assessment of patients' competence to consent to treatment. *N Engl J Med.* 2007; 357:1834–1840.

3. Wood JM, Anstey KJ, Kerr GK, Lacherez PF, Lords S. A multidomain approach for predicting older driver safety under in-traffic road conditions. *J Am Geriatr Soc.* 2008;56:986–993.

4. Lyketsos CG, Lopez O, Jones B, Fitzpatrick AL, Breitner J, DeKosky S. Prevalence of neuropsychiatric symptoms in dementia and mild cognitive impairment. *JAMA.* 2002;288:1475–1483.

5. Bruera E, Neumann CM. Management of specific symptom complexes in patients receiving palliative care. *CMAJ.* 1998;158(13):1717–1726.

6. Ball K, Berch DB, Helmers KF, et al. Effects of cognitive training interventions with older adults. *JAMA.* 2002;288:2271–2281.

7. Lautenschlager NT, Cox KL, Flicker L, et al. Effect of physical activity on cognitive function in older adults at risk for Alzheimer's disease. *JAMA.* 2008;300:1027–1037.

8. Verghese J, Lipton RB, Katz MJ, et al. Leisure activities and the risk of dementia in the elderly. *N Engl J Med.* 2003;19:2508–2516.

9. Qaseem A, Snow V, Cross T, et al. Current pharmacologic treatment of dementia: a clinical practice guideline from the American College of Physicians and the American Academy of Family Physicians. *Ann Intern Med.* 2008;148:370–378.

10. *American Medical Association Diagnostic and Treatment Guidelines on Elder Abuse and Neglect.* Chicago, IL: American Medical Association; 1992.

11. Fulmer T, Guadagno L, Bitondo Dyer C, et al. Progress in elder abuse screening and assessment instruments. *J Am Geriatr Soc.* 2004;52:297–304.

12. Lachs MS, Pillemer K. Abuse and neglect of elderly persons. *N Engl J Med.* 1995;332:437–443.

CHAPTER THIRTY

Addressing Health Literacy in Geriatric Outpatient Practices

Michael S. Wolf, PhD, MPH

Alex Federman, MD, MPH

MR BEACH'S EXPERIENCE

Mr Beach is a 72-year-old man with a history of long-standing hypertension and hyperlipidemia who was recently diagnosed with type II diabetes mellitus. A trial of lifestyle modification failed to adequately control his hyperglycemia, so a decision was made to start glyburide, 5 mg twice a day. His physician tells him why the drug is important and a bit about how it works. She then explains how to take the medication, saying "take one tablet twice a day before meals."

At his follow-up visit a few months later, the physician finds that Mr Beach's glycemia has not improved. The physician learns that Mr Beach stopped taking the medication more than a month ago because it was making his sugar too low, causing him to feel ill. On further questioning, Mr Beach reveals that he was taking the glyburide before *all* meals, including snacks, up to 25 mg a day.

INTRODUCTION

Health literacy is the degree to which individuals have the capacity to obtain, process, and understand basic health information and services needed to make appropriate health decisions.[1]

Health literacy represents a set of skills that enable individuals to process health-related information to successfully perform health care–related tasks, make informed decisions, and navigate various health systems. It is a multifaceted concept, of which both reading and numeracy skills are fundamental components. During the past two decades, a large body of evidence has linked measures of reading and numeracy skills to chronic disease outcomes, risk of hospitalization, and mortality. This has led clinicians and policy makers to cite health literacy as a major clinical and public health issue.

Health literacy is a particularly important issue for older adults because of its association with cognitive function. Research shows that health literacy is strongly related to cognition.[1] Individuals must apply a constellation of cognitive abilities to register and process health information, including short- and long-term memory, concentration, and interpretive and inferential skills, among others. Processing speed, which declines with age, is another aspect of cognition that plays an important role in patients' ability to work with health information.

The patient, Mr Beach, had to sort through the information from his physician about glyburide (its importance, how it works, how to take it), identify the most important information (how to take it), and infer when exactly to take the pills. This cognitive process occurred in the context of a physician-patient encounter, but the same challenges for the patient could have arisen with any modality of information transfer, including print materials, video messages, the Internet, and telephone. For instance, the patient had the prescription bottle at home and had the opportunity to read the instructions on the label. However, instructions on standard prescription labels often require patients to interpret how or when to take the medications, and they frequently misinterpret the information.[2]

As this case and recent research illustrates, cognitive function must be considered when communicating health information to patients—that is, when addressing health literacy—especially in older adults.

OPPORTUNITIES

Patients are generally expected to engage in their own health care and execute the recommendations and prescriptions of their health care providers. But the health care system, including individual health care providers, has a greater responsibility to ensure that patients are able to meet the demands that accompany engagement in health care. Health care providers can reach this end by promoting health literacy. This chapter identifies opportunities and specific tools to meet the health literacy needs of older adults in outpatient clinical settings.

Opportunities to address health literacy limitations arise at all occasions in which information is transferred to patients. This includes print, verbal, and multimedia communications. In this chapter we highlight some of the situations in which communication appropriately tailored to the patient's health literacy skills may have a particularly meaningful impact on self-management and health outcomes.

Promoting health literacy means helping individuals better comprehend health information, make appropriate decisions, and ultimately take action. While writing materials at lower grade levels is one part of addressing health literacy limitations, other general strategies are usually needed as well. These include (1) improving the clarity of print materials, (2) improving the clarity of verbal communication, (3) considering cognitive limitations, and (4) reinforcing learning.

1. Improve the clarity of print materials.

➤ Simplify print materials for easy understandability across all literacy levels. (See Table 30-1 for specific recommendations and the Useful Resources section at the end of this chapter for Web-based resources)

  ➤ Write in large font.

  ➤ Use plain language and avoid medical jargon.

  ➤ Make sentences brief and focused on a single concept.

  ➤ Make sentences action-oriented.

➤ Use visual aids—this facilitates information retention and processing, especially for complex concepts.

  ➤ Figures or images should be simple, recognizable, and clear.

  ➤ Tailor visual aids to reflect the culture, age, and background of the patient population.

  ➤ Photographs and visual materials depicting how to correctly engage in health activities can be very effective methods of delivering health information.

  ➤ See the Useful Resources section for Web-based resources that provide low-literacy educational materials or guide their design.

TABLE 30-1 Techniques to Improve Understandability of Written Materials

Technique	Explanation
Write in short sentences	Short sentences tend to be easier for patients to read and understand. Sentence length should be less than 15 words and ideally less than 10 words. Sentences should be written in a conversational style.
Print in large, sans-serif font	Text should be written in sans-serif font (eg, Arial) with a minimum font size of 12 pt. Use of all-capital letters should be avoided; only the first letter of words in sentences should be capitalized.
Include sufficient white space	Large margins and adequate spacing between sentences and paragraphs will provide sufficient white space and prevent a document from appearing to be solid text. In general, text should be left-justified for easy reading.
Select simple words	Words that are commonly used in conversation are the best to include in health messages. Shorter words tend to be easier to understand and more familiar to patients.
Provide information in bulleted lists	Bullets help to separate information from the rest of the text. Information provided in lists is often easier and faster for patients to read and comprehend.
Highlight or underline key information	Using boldface and highlighting phrases or words can draw attention to essential information for patients. It should be used sparingly to differentiate key sentences or phrases from the rest of the text.
Design passages to be action- and goal-oriented	Written passages should be action- and goal-oriented and should provide readers with a clear explanation of the purpose of the written material. Passages should clearly define what actions should be taken by the reader and why these actions are necessary.
Group and limit instructional content	Consider grouping information under common headings to promote understanding. Place key information in the beginning of a paragraph, and be sure to limit the amount of instructional content that is given to what is essential for the patient to know and understand.
Use active voice	Information written in the active voice is easier to understand and more likely to motivate the patient to action.
Avoid unnecessary jargon	Unnecessary jargon can be distracting to patients and often provides little information. Medical terminology should be used as infrequently as possible and, if used, should always be clearly defined and explained to the patient.

2. Improve verbal communication.

➤ Always use plain language when speaking with patients; avoid use of medical jargon.[3]

➤ Define and clarify medical terms and concepts.

➤ Speak clearly and listen carefully.

➤ Prompt with open-ended, rather than yes-no, questions.

  ➤ Ask questions using the words "what" or "how" instead of those that can be answered with "yes" or "no."

  ➤ For example, "Tell me about your problem. What may have caused it?"

  ➤ Try asking "What questions do you have?" instead of "Do you have any questions?"

➤ Make information specific to the goal for behavior.

  ➤ Teach-to-goal: directly counsel toward the specific goal and avoid use of distracting information.[4]

➤ Allow sufficient time for the patient to register and process verbal information.

➤ Verify understanding by using "teach-back" or guided imagery.

  ➤ Teach-back technique[5]:

    ➤ The health care clinician asks the patient to reiterate the information just discussed, focusing on one or two of the main points.

    ➤ If the patient's recall is incorrect, the health care clinician reviews the information and gives the patient another opportunity to demonstrate understanding.

    ➤ This process ensures that the patient has adequately understood the information.

    ➤ Teach-back is an important patient safety technique.[6]

  ➤ Guided imagery[7]:

    ➤ Patients are asked to explicitly describe how they will perform a recommended behavior (eg, medication use).

    ➤ Examples: what time of day they will take a medicine, where they will store the medicine, how they will remind themselves to perform a specific health-related task, the specific situation in which blood glucose level will be checked and how it will be checked.

3. Consider cognitive impairment.

Mild cognitive impairment is present in up to 17% of the elderly US population and may not be apparent to the health care clinician.[8] Early deficits in cognitive function include working memory, processing speed, and executive function (task-oriented cognitive abilities).

➤ Communication should be directed toward older patients with an awareness of potential cognitive deficits.

➤ *Working memory:* Limit the burden on working memory by providing the most salient, goal-oriented health information; repeat and reinforce information. Try to convey no more than four or five new pieces of information at a time.

➤ *Processing speed:* Allow sufficient time for patients to consider health information.

➤ *Executive function:* Present information in discrete, single-concept units; be concrete and specific—do not present information that requires the patient to draw inferences.

   ➤ For example, tell patients precisely how many hours after dinner to check their blood glucose, rather than simply telling them to check it "after dinner."

4. Reinforce learning.

➤ Use teach-back as described above.

➤ Provide tangible, print materials to accompany verbally communicated information.

➤ Use multimedia strategies when possible (printed instructions with illustrations and figures, video).

➤ Repeat messages often.

CHALLENGES

1. Health literacy measurement.

➤ There are no efficient tools for assessing health literacy in clinical practice.

➤ Screening could introduce feelings of shame or embarrassment.

➤ Routine health literacy screening in clinical care is not recommended.

2. Time.

➤ Time is needed to acquire or create low-literacy health information materials.

➤ Ensuring that patients understand health information can add time to clinical encounters.

3. Skills development.

➤ Health care clinicians need to develop specific skills for communicating effectively with patients.

➤ Specific skills are required to make health information materials comprehensible for low-literacy and elderly patients.

SOLUTIONS

1. Office staff training and communication skills.

➤ Train staff to have an attitude of helpfulness.

> ➤ People with low health literacy often feel embarrassed or stigmatized, which may prevent them from seeking help or clarification of information they do not understand.

> ➤ Staff should strive to mitigate low-literacy patients' fears by proactively offering assistance.

> ➤ They should offer all patients assistance with completion of health and insurance forms.

> ➤ They should provide simplified explanations of office procedures.

> ➤ Because low-literacy patients can be difficult to identify, staff should take these approaches with all patients.

➤ Scheduling appointments

> ➤ Avoid use of automated phone trees.

> ➤ Staff should offer to provide directions.

> ➤ Instruct patients to bring in their medications and a list of questions they might have for the physician.

➤ Forms and paperwork

> ➤ Forms should be easy to read and written in the patient's language.

➤ Forms should collect only essential information.

➤ Staff should offer assistance completing forms.

➤ Additional information about how to make your office patient-friendly can be found in the AMA Foundation publication, *Health Literacy and Patient Safety: Help Your Patients Understand*[6]

2. Addressing measurement barriers.

➤ Avoid screening or assessing for health literacy; rather, simplify health information for all patients.

➤ Identify patients who may need additional support; following are some clues:

　➤ Patient has less than a high school graduate level of education or is socioeconomically disadvantaged

　➤ Paperwork is left incomplete

　➤ Patient refuses to complete a form, perhaps saying he or she has forgotten reading glasses

➤ Ask patients about problems with reading and comprehension when you suspect a problem, but expect that patients with low literacy may experience feelings of shame or may have concerns about stigma.

　➤ Use simple, direct questions to alleviate much of the shame and stigma a patient may feel with regard to reading and writing limitations.

　　➤ "How often do you have any trouble reading printed forms?"

　　➤ "How often do you have someone help you read health materials?"

　　➤ If the patient responds affirmatively, health care providers may need to spend additional time with the patient reviewing pertinent health information and verifying that the patient understands the information presented.

3. Time-saving measures.

➤ Apply the focused counseling strategies discussed in Chapter 31, Self-management Support for Older Adults.

➤ Realize that time spent on clarification of health information may save time during future encounters by avoiding the need for extensive review of information or correcting errors.

➤ Use existing health literacy materials. A number of useful Web-based resources are listed in the Useful Resources section.

4. Developing basic skills for clear health communication.

➤ This is simple and quick and is important for all staff in the office who interact with patients.

  ➤ Eliminate jargon.

  ➤ Teach to goal.

  ➤ Assess comprehension by using the teach-back method.

ADDRESSING THE HEALTH LITERACY ISSUES FACING MR BEACH

The experience of Mr Beach is not unique. He, along with 29% of adults age 65 or greater have less than basic health literacy skills and an additional 30% have basic literacy skills and are prone to medical errors and problems of "adherence."[9, 10] Nearly half of older patients misunderstand seemingly simple prescription medication labeling.[2] By applying the concepts described above, the physician might have helped avert the Mr Beach's hypoglycemic episodes and subsequent medication nonadherence. For example, the physician could have:

➤ Identified in advance the most important information the patient needed

➤ Eliminated discussion of distracting information, such as how the medication works

➤ Used a teach-to-goal strategy, focusing exclusively on how to use the medication

➤ Used teach-back to ensure comprehension of the plan

➤ Made the information more concrete by linking the usage time to specific times of day, such as meal times or specific hours of the day (see Table 30-1 for specific examples)[11]

➤ Provided the patient with written, simplified instructions on how to use the medications

  ➤ List the purpose of the medication, its name (including generic name if a branded drug is prescribed) and dose, frequency of administration, and when to take it.

Box 30-1 Example of Simplified Medication Use Instructions for Patients

For your high blood pressure:

1. Prinivil, 40 mg (this drug is also sometimes called lisinopril)

    Take 1 tablet every day.

    Take it with breakfast.

2. Metoprolol, 50 mg

    Take 1 tablet twice a day.

    Take 1 tablet with breakfast and 1 tablet with dinner.

TAKE-HOME POINTS

➤ Low health literacy is highly prevalent, especially in older populations.

➤ Improve understanding of health information by using plain language, accounting for possible cognitive impairment, using a teach-to-goal strategy, and confirming understanding by applying the teach-back method.

➤ Provide written, well-designed, and simple take-home materials to reinforce and support information communicated verbally or through video.

USEFUL RESOURCES

AMA Foundation

➤ *Health Literacy and Patient Safety: Help Patients Understand* (www.ama-assn.org/ama1/pub/upload/mm/367/healthlitclinicians.pdf).

➤ A manual for clinicians for making office practices user-friendly to patients with limited literacy; includes case-based studies and video demonstrations.

U.S. Agency for Health care Research and Quality

➤ *Quick Guide to Health Literacy* (www.health.gov/communication/literacy/quickguide/Quickguide.pdf).

➤ Describes health literacy and provides examples of plain language for written materials and verbal communication.

US Government

➤ (www.plainlanguage.gov/).

➤ Explanations and examples of plain language for written materials and verbal communication.

US Food and Drug Administration

➤ (http://discoveryhealthcme.discovery.com/risk/risk.html).

➤ Web-based video tutorial on discussing risk with patients, with strategies for low-literacy patients.

Low-Literacy Patient Education Materials

Healthy Roads (funded by the National Cancer Institute)

➤ (www.healthyroadsmedia.org/).

➤ Materials available in different formats (paper, Web, video, audio) on various health topics.

National Library of Medicine/National Institutes of Health

➤ (www.nlm.nih.gov/medlineplus/easytoread/easytoread_a.html).

➤ Very large collection of low-literacy educational material on a broad range of chronic illnesses and other health related issues; includes paper, Web, and interactive Web-based materials.

Health Literacy Interventions

Canadian Public Health Association

➤ Health Literacy Interventions (www.cpha.ca/uploads/Portals/h-l/interventions_e.pdf).

➤ Includes examples of how to address specific clinical issues with low-literacy patients, such as diabetes management, and counseling on cancer screening.

Information Clearinghouses

California Health Literacy Initiative

➤ (http://cahealthliteracy.org/rc/12.html).

➤ Links to programs that address literacy issues for different chronic conditions.

Harvard School of Public Health

➤ (www.hsph.harvard.edu/healthliteracy/index.html).

➤ Includes information on interventions as well as information on health literacy research.

US Department of Health and Human Services

➤ (www.health.gov/communication/literacy/quickguide/resources.htm).

➤ Links to various tools for improving or testing readability of written materials.

REFERENCES

1. Institute of Medicine; Nielsen-Bohlman L, Panzer A, Kindig DA, eds. *Health Literacy: A Prescription to End Confusion.* Washington, DC: National Academies Press; 2004.

2. Davis TC, Wolf MS, Bass PF III, et al. Literacy and misunderstanding prescription drug labels. *Ann Intern Med.* 2006;145(12):887–894.

3. Paasche-Orlow MK, Schillinger D, Greene SM, Wagner EH. How health care systems can begin to address the challenge of limited literacy. *J Gen Intern Med.* 2006;21(8):884–887.

4. DeWalt DA, Broucksou KA, Hawk V, et al. Comparison of a one-time educational intervention to a teach-to-goal educational intervention for self-management of heart failure: design of a randomized controlled trial. *BMC Health Serv Res.* 2009;9:99.

5. Schillinger D, Piette J, Grumbach K, et al. Closing the loop: physician communication with diabetic patients who have low health literacy. *Arch Intern Med.* 2003;163:83–90.

6. AMA Foundation. *Health Literacy and Patient Safety: Help Patients Understand.* 2007. Available at: www.ama-assn.org/ama1/pub/upload/mm/367/healthlitclinicians.pdf.

7. Park DC, Gutchess AH, Meade ML, Stine-Morrow EA. Improving cognitive function in older adults: nontraditional approaches. *J Gerontol.* 2007;62B:45–52.

8. Mariani E, Monastero R, Mecocci P. Mild cognitive impairment: a systematic review. *J Alzheimers Dis.* 2007;12(1):23–35.

9. Centers for Disease Control and Prevention, Improving Health Literacy for Older Adults: Expert Panel Report 2009 Atlanta: US Department of Health and Human Services; 2009.

10. Kutner M, Greenberg E, Jin Y, Paulsen C. The Health Literacy of America's Adults: Results from the 2003 National Assessment of Adult Literacy. Washington DC: US department of Education, National Center for Education Statistics; 2006. Publication no. 2006–483.

11. Davis TC, Federman AD, Bass PF, et al. Improving patient understanding of prescription drug instructions. *J Gen Intern Med.* 2009;24:57–62.

CHAPTER | THIRTY-ONE

Self-management Support for Older Adults

Connie L. Davis, GNP, BC

John H. Wasson, MD

MRS SHELBY'S EXPERIENCE

Mrs Shelby, a 79-year-old patient with diabetes, heart failure, hypertension, and arthritis, returns to your office for a routine follow-up. She has had multiple hospital admissions for heart failure. You have spent time teaching her to monitor her symptoms and weight and to call you for directions when this happens, but she has gone to the hospital instead. You are also puzzled to find that her blood pressure is not under better control at this visit. You had added a second antihypertensive on her last visit. Mrs Shelby is accompanied by her son and they tell you that they heard what you said about monitoring weight and symptoms, but when she is at home Mrs Shelby does not seem to know what she is supposed to do, so she wants to go to the emergency department whenever she can't "catch her breath."

OPPORTUNITIES

To achieve positive health outcomes, patients and caregivers must correctly apply the self-management regimens prescribed by their physicians. However, as with Mrs Shelby, even the simplest of tasks can be challenging for older patients. Patients often have difficulty understanding the information given them by physicians, struggle with problem solving, have beliefs about their medications and illness that adversely affect their self-management, and often experience limited confidence in managing their health.[1]

The clinical encounter presents physicians with the opportunity to bolster their patients' self-management skills and promote better health outcomes. When properly planned, communicating with patients outside of the clinical setting, such as by e-mail or telephone, and doing so with nonphysician staff has also proved to be very effective.[2]

Assessing and Facilitating Patient Understanding

Understanding the information presented is a prerequisite for taking action. *Health literacy* encapsulates the set of skills that patients need to understand and act on health information. Approximately one third of adults 65 years or older lack basic health literacy skills to successfully navigate the health care system and make health care decisions.[3, 4] Chapter 30, Addressing Health Literacy in Geriatric Outpatient Practices, details how physicians can improve older patients' understanding of health information.

Practicing Patient-Centered Care

Patient-centered care is at the core of successful promotion of good self-management. The Institute of Medicine has cited patient-centered care as a key element in improving and maintaining quality, and identifies it as encompassing "qualities of compassion, empathy, and responsiveness to the needs, values, and expressed preferences of the individual patient."[5] Strategies to support patient-centered care include collaborative decision making and problem solving; the establishment of clear, measurable health goals; and formation of meaningful, realistic plans to attain the goals.[6]

Support of Self-management

Three robust assumptions undergird self-management strategies for patients across a range of conditions.[7] First, different chronic conditions present similar self-management problems to patients. Second, patients can usually take responsibility for the day-to-day management of most chronic conditions. Third, confident patients practicing self-management will generally experience improved health status. Therefore, the most effective strategies physicians and members of a health care team use to support their patients have commonalities,[8] including (1) identification of the self-management objectives that matter to the patient; (2) a clearly defined plan; (3) the use of problem solving and teaching to support the plan; and (4) repeated reinforcement of the previous three steps.

Assessing patients' confidence in their ability to carry out self-management tasks is a useful way to monitor and positively reinforce their chronic disease self-management. For example, after inquiring about their confidence, their physician learned that Mrs Shelby and her son had not recognized the nexus among the physiologic measures of weight and blood pressure and her symptom of "shortness of breath." The physician could have assessed their confidence to manage her congestive heart failure self-monitoring tasks by asking, "How confident are you that you can check your weight every day?" This approach would have allowed Mrs Shelby, her son, and the physician the opportunity to correct their divergent objectives and plans.

The following checklist of supportive actions for self-management might also have proved useful to the physician.

A. Identify objectives

    1. Engage the patient in identifying treatment goals and self-management strategies

    2. Focus on behavior-related tasks

B. Define the plan

    1. Make the plan specific and concrete: when, where, how, how often

    2. Recognize that the physician is often not the best person to be central to the plan. Other health professionals, peers, and family are often crucial for the success of the plan

C. Problem solve

    1. Work with patients to identify barriers to self-management goals

    2. Develop patient-centered problem-solving strategies

        a. Ask what they think might help them overcome the barriers

        b. Help them arrive at their own solutions

D. Teach

    1. Focus teaching on the main objectives (teach-to-goal; see Chapter 30)

    2. Tailor information to the patient's cultural background (see Chapter 32)

    3. Consider health literacy limitations

    4. Probe patients' beliefs about illness and medications, and correct erroneous beliefs

        a. What are the symptoms of the illness or medication?

        b. What causes the illness?

      c.   What effect does the medication have on the illness?

      d.   How long will they have the illness?

      e.   How long will they need to continue the treatment?

      f.   What would happen if they stopped a treatment?

      g.   Can their condition be controlled or cured?

E. Reinforce

    1.   Provide a written summary of the goals, strategies, and expectations

    2.   Assess and reassess the patient's progress toward the identified goal

    3.   Provide concrete feedback on performance

    4.   Provide encouragement

    5.   Readdress the goals, strategies, and learning over multiple encounters

    6.   Assess and monitor confidence with self-management

ANTICIPATED RESULTS

Improving patients' understanding of health information and providing patient-centered self-management support can result in a number of positive outcomes including the following[9]:

➤ Improved patient and caregiver confidence with self-management

➤ Improved medication adherence and self-monitoring

➤ Improved chronic disease control

➤ Reduced use of acute care services, like hospitalization and emergency department care

➤ Improved patient and provider satisfaction

➤ Stronger patient-provider relationships

CHALLENGES

Beyond a lack of understanding, a variety of patient factors can adversely affect success with self-management, including inadequate problem-solving skills, inappropriate beliefs about illness and medications, and patients' lack of confidence in their ability to self-manage.

Health system barriers to effectively support self-management include the perception that additional time will be needed to counsel patients on self-management strategies, a lack of self-management support skills among physicians and staff, and the lack of a system to build self-management into office practice.

SOLUTIONS AND RESOURCES

Time-saving solutions: Problem solving and action planning can often be completed in 5 minutes.

- Brief, focused counseling

  - Teach-to-goal: direct counseling toward the specific goal and avoid use of distracting information; see also Chapter 30

- Automated follow-up, monitoring, and reinforcement of goals/teaching

  - Automated telephone follow-up is an effective method for promoting self-management behaviors

  - Routine face-to-face and electronic follow-up can also be built into clinical practices. See the AMA's Physician Resource Guide to Patient Self-management Support (www.ama-assn.org/ama1/pub/upload/mm/433/phys_resource_guide.pdf).

- Use of nonphysician staff to help deliver self-management support (in person, by telephone, or by e-mail)

- Steps to getting started, with specific examples:

  - Patient and physician agree on a self-management goal to complete before the next visit

    - Mrs Shelby and her son agree the goal is to prevent increasing shortness of breath.

  - Establish a plan to achieve the goal.

    - The son will monitor weight and adjust the furosemide dosage when weight change is more than 3 pounds.

  - Make the plan specific and concrete: when, where, how, how often

> ➤ A practice team member and Mrs Shelby's son will touch base every 3 days initially, and then weekly if all goes well.

➤ Problem-solve to overcome patient-perceived barriers to reaching the goal (see detail below)

> ➤ The patient's son and the nurse establish an e-mail contact method for questions.

➤ Assess confidence

> ➤ A practice team member and the physician assess the patient's and son's confidence with this plan, problem-solve for issues where confidence is low, and reassess confidence on e-mail contacts

➤ Provide written instructions

➤ Have the patient follow up with the physician in 6 weeks

> ➤ Assess their progress and reinforce learning

> ➤ Problem-solve (for example, blood pressure control, if still needed)

> ➤ Offer encouragement

Resources for self-management support training for health care professionals:

➤ Primer for conducting brief personal action planning with patients

> ➤ www.ama-assn.org/ama1/pub/upload/mm/433/ub_pap.pdf

➤ Physician tip sheet for self-management support

> ➤ www.ama-assn.org/ama1/pub/upload/mm/433/phys_tip_sheet.pdf

➤ Video demonstrating self-management support

> ➤ www.chcf.org/publications/2008/08/video-on-coaching-patients-for-successful-selfmanagement

Introduce patients to self-management support tools they can access themselves:

➤ Web-based resources

> ➤ From Dartmouth Medical School, http://howsyourhealth.org/ and http://decisionsinthegrey.org.

➤ The Stanford University School of Medicine has a number of self-management and patient education materials, available for purchase: http://patienteducation.stanford.edu/materials/

➤ Be aware of community resources for older adults, generally accessed through the local Area Agency on Aging. Local programs can be located through www.aoa.gov/

TAKE-HOME POINTS

➤ Effective self-management is rooted in the concept of patient-centered care

➤ Work with patients to identify treatment goals and strategies to meet the goals

➤ Make self-management plans concrete

➤ Be aware of health literacy limitations and cultural factors

➤ Monitor progress and reinforce learning

➤ Assess patients' confidence in their ability to carry out a plan to identify topics that need additional problem-solving and encouragement

➤ When possible, use nonphysician staff to help support self-management

➤ After testing, integrate the most effective strategies into your practice's normal workflow

USEFUL RESOURCES

California Health Care Foundation

Useful resources for supporting patient self-management in clinical practices (www.chcf.org/publications/2009/09/selfmanagement-support-training-materials).

American Medical Association

➤ Physician Resource Guide to Patient Self-management Support (www.ama-assn.org/ama1/pub/upload/mm/433/phys_resource_guide.pdf).

Robert Wood Johnson Foundation

➤ Concepts about diabetes self-management support that can be applied to self-management of other chronic diseases (http://diabetesnpo.im.wustl.edu/).

DeWalt DA, Broucksou KA, Hawk V, et al. Comparison of a one-time educational intervention to a teach-to-goal educational intervention for self-management of heart failure: design of a randomized controlled trial. *BMC Health Serv Res*. 2009;9:99.

Handley MA, Shumway M, Schillinger D. Cost-effectiveness of automated telephone self-management support with nurse care management among patients with diabetes. *Ann Fam Med*. 2008;6(6):512–518.

McAndrew LM, Musumeci-Szabó TJ, Mora PA, et al. Using the common sense model to design interventions for the prevention and management of chronic illness threats: from description to process. *Br J Health Psychol*. 2008;13(pt 2):195–204.

REFERENCES

1. Harrington J, Noble LM, Newman SP. Improving patients' communication with doctors: a systematic review of intervention studies. *Patient Educ Couns.* 2004;52(1):7–16.

2. Ahles TA, Wasson JW, Seville JL, et al. A controlled trial of methods for managing pain in primary care patients with or without co-occurring psychosocial problems. *Ann Fam Med.* 2006;4(3):341–350.

3. Centers for Disease Control and Prevention, Improving Health Literacy for Older Adults: Expert Panel Report 2009 Atlanta: US Department of Health and Human Services; 2009.

4. Kutner M, Greenberg E, Jin Y, Paulsen C. The Health Literacy of America's Adults: Results from the 2003 National Assessment of Adult Literacy. Washington DC: US department of Education, National Center for Education Statistics; 2006. Publication no. 2006–483.

5. Institute of Medicine. *Crossing the Quality Chasm: A New Health System for the 21st Century.* Washington, DC: National Academies Press; 2009.

6. Wagner EH, Austin BT, VonKorff MV. Optimizing care for patients with chronic illness. *Milbank Q.* 1996;74(4):511–542.

7. Lorig KR, Sobel DS, Stewart AL, et al. Evidence suggesting that a chronic disease self-management program can improve health status while reducing hospitalization: a randomized trial. *Med Care.* 1999;37(1):5–14.

8. Glazier RH, Bajcar J, Kennie NR, et al. Meta-analysis: chronic disease self-management programs for older adults. A systematic review of interventions to improve diabetes care in socially disadvantaged populations. *Diabetes Care.* 2006;29(7):1675–1688.

9. American Medical Association. Physician Resource Guide to Self-management Support. Available at: www.ama-assn.org/ama1/pub/upload/mm/433/phys_resource_guide.pdf.

CHAPTER | THIRTY-TWO

Culturally Effective Care and Health Disparity

Arun S. Rao, MD

Seema Limaye, MD

PATIENT EXPERIENCES

An 89-year-old woman comes into the office for the evaluation of a rash and agitation at home. She is unable to provide a detailed history but is accompanied by her Filipino home health aide, who speaks English but who clearly has difficulty communicating with you and understanding your instructions. You decide to write down some of the basic points in simple English and to provide appropriate written educational materials with the assistance of an interpreter.

A 67-year-old Puerto Rican Spanish-speaking woman is evaluated for intractable pain from metastatic breast cancer. Her oncologist, having difficulty communicating with her, continues to give her treatments that are clearly causing her physical and emotional distress. Finally, by using interpreter services, it becomes clear that she wants no further therapies and prefers instead to enroll in a hospice program and live out her final days with her family. Following this discussion, her pain and emotional distress are noticeably diminished.

An 87-year-old Farsi-speaking Pakistani man is seen in follow-up for complications of his transfusion-dependent myelodysplastic syndrome. Your office staff is frustrated because he and his family do not speak English and repeatedly confuse appointments, billing issues, and instructions for follow-up. His condition is progressing and his prognosis is poor. He has had trouble expressing symptoms and goals to you, and you are becoming frustrated as well. You decide to hold a family meeting to address some of these issues. During this meeting, it becomes clear that there are many cultural and medical issues that need to be addressed on all parties' sides before proceeding with his care.

BACKGROUND INFORMATION

Good communication is at the heart of every good relationship between physicians and patients.[1] These vignettes highlight some of the common problems encountered by physicians, patients, and caregivers in communicating with older adults from different ethnic and cultural backgrounds as well as across language barriers. They also point to the important role of understanding cross-cultural communication and knowing what resources are available to assist health care providers (HCPs), medical office staff, patients, and their families/caregivers.

Nationwide, older adults compose 12% of the overall population and ethnic minorities make up 16% of the population older than 65 years. This latter number is expected to rise to 25% to 30% by 2050, highlighting a need for health care providers and staff to be aware of cross-cultural issues in patient care[2]. Patients from ethnic minority groups traditionally have higher burdens of medical illness, poorer access to care, higher rates of dissatisfaction with health care, and inferior comprehension of their health and treatments, leading to poorer health outcomes[3-5]. Furthermore, limited English proficiency has been cited as one of the major barriers to accessing health care for minorities and older adults. Other difficult issues in communicating with older adults such as limited time, poor reimbursement, ageist attitudes and biases, patient embarrassment, sensory and cognitive impairments, low rates of health literacy, and third-party informants highlight why initiatives to improve communication between HCPs and older ethnic adults will be so critical in the coming years[6]. Research robustly links better communication between patients and medical caregivers to enhanced medical adherence, satisfaction with care, appropriate utilization of services, physicians' ability to diagnose and treat, physician satisfaction, fewer malpractice suits, and overall improved medical outcomes.[7] Studies in adult and pediatric populations have demonstrated that the use of medical interpreters improves patient satisfaction with care and physicians, adherence with medical recommendations, and understanding of medical discussions, and reduces the stress levels of HCPs caring for patients with limited English proficiency.[7]

Important Terms in Cross-Cultural Care

➤ Race

   ➤ Anthropological categories of people

   ➤ Traditionally differentiated on basis of inheritable physical characteristics

   ➤ Social construct

➤ Culture

   ➤ A shared system of knowledge, beliefs, values, attitudes, and learned patterns of behavior

➤ Ethnicity

> ➤ Subgroups of people who share ancestry, history, or culture

> ➤ Often associated with geography and language/dialect

> ➤ Influential in culture, religion, and gender roles

➤ Acculturation

> ➤ Process by which members of one cultural group adopt beliefs and values of another

➤ Limited English proficiency

> ➤ Limited ability to read, write, speak, or understand English

> ➤ Often a barrier to accessing important benefits or services, understanding and exercising important rights, complying with applicable responsibilities, or understanding other information provided by federally funded programs and activities

Important Topics in Caring for Older Adults From Different Backgrounds

➤ *Awareness of changing demographics:*

> ➤ Ethnic/minority older population increasing in size[5]

> > ➤ Estimated to be 25% to 30% of US population older than 65 years by 2050

> ➤ Ethnic/minority representation in health care

> > ➤ 11% of total US physicians[5]

> > ➤ Some ethnic/racial groups are overrepresented in medical field compared with general population

> > ➤ Potential for cultural discordance, misunderstandings, miscommunication

➤ *Conducting a culturally sensitive history and physical examination:*

> ➤ Appreciate cultural, ethnic, and historical backgrounds, but *individualize* all aspects of the encounter.

> ➤ Elucidate patient's preferred term for his/her cultural identity.

> ➤ Elucidate patient's preferred method of being addressed.

> > ➤ Always start formally (eg, title + surname).

> > ➤ Pay attention to pronunciation.

➤ Be aware of the role of family members/friends.

  ➤ Decision-making roles

  ➤ Diagnosis/prognosis disclosure issues

➤ Be aware of body positioning, body language, hand gesturing, facial expressions, physical and eye contact.

  ➤ Try to start more formally/conservatively.

  ➤ Try to avoid expressive extremes.

  ➤ Some cultures prohibit direct eye contact between people of different levels of authority or different genders; do not interpret lack of eye contact as distraction or disinterest.

➤ *Language and health literacy:*

  ➤ Elucidate patient's preferred language.

  ➤ Assess health literacy tactfully.

    ➤ Avoid shame and potentially shaming situations such as:

      ➤ Asking "What things do you like to read?"

      ➤ Asking "How far did you go in school?"

      ➤ Asking the patient to read a prescription bottle.

  ➤ Use plain language.

  ➤ Slow down.

  ➤ Use repetition and "teach-back" techniques.

  ➤ Demonstrate or draw pictures.

  ➤ Limit information.

  ➤ Be respectful, caring, and sensitive.

➤ *Office/setting should be navigable to patients:*

  ➤ Appointment/telephone service: support staff should be trained to determine when telephone-based interpreter services are appropriate and how to conference a patient call with the service.

  ➤ Signs should be in appropriate languages: registration, pharmacy, laboratory, testing.

  ➤ Forms should be available in appropriate languages: insurance, registration questionnaires.

  ➤ Patient education materials/handouts should be available in appropriate languages.

> ➤ Hours when care is provided should be convenient and appropriate to patients' needs and life situations.

➤ *Tools/resources to facilitate communication if language discordance exists (see Table 32-1):*

> ➤ Pacific Interpreters (telephone; fee)
>
> > ➤ www.pacificinterpreters.com/
>
> ➤ AT&T Language Line (telephone; fee)
>
> > ➤ www.languageline.com/page/industry_healthcare/

TABLE 32-1 Interpreter Strengths and Weaknesses

Type of Interpreter	Description	Strengths	Limitations
Professional interpreters on staff	Institution/agency employed and trained; usually available for languages most frequently encountered at institution	Available during operating hours; interpreters are trained professionally and experienced	Costly for the institution; may not be available off-hours; may not cover all languages needed; often need to prearrange or schedule
On-call interpreters	May be paid/volunteer; list maintained by agency/institution	Similar to above; may cover broader variety of languages	Training may vary depending on institution's requirements; availability may be limited; emergencies may pose problem
Bilingual staff	Health care staff or support staff	Availability; usually no associated cost	Individual training as an interpreter; unfamiliar with specialized terminology/vocabulary; potential conflict in duties/roles/responsibilities
Family, children, friends	Usually accompany patient	Availability	Untrained, unfamiliar with medical terminology/vocabulary; documented in literature to make frequent errors; potential to interfere with family dynamics, confidentiality, and other relationships; children are never appropriate unless emergency
Telephone service (eg, Pacific Interpreting Services or AT&T Language Line)	Over-the-telephone interpretation; available by subscription to agency/institution	Availability; rapid access; broad spectrum of languages and dialects covered; interpreters are native speakers with training in specialized terminology	Speakerphone best; hearing/cognitively impaired patients have trouble; costly; mental health issues

➤ Internet-based translator tools

   ➤ For example, Google Translator (free)

      ➤ www.google.com/language_tools?hl=en

   ➤ Most are free

   ➤ Translation is usually verbatim, can be inaccurate

   ➤ Sometimes translated into different scripts that either physician or patient cannot read

➤ Hospital, institutional, community interpreter, and translator services

➤ *Knowledge of patients' cultural backgrounds/history:*

   ➤ Be aware of subtle cultural "subgroups" rather than usual stereotypes

      ➤ For example, Spanish is a language, not a culture

      ➤ For example, African American/black patients have varied backgrounds and cultural roots

         ➤ Caribbean

         ➤ African

         ➤ American

➤ *Other factors to consider:*

   ➤ Trust in health care system

   ➤ Immigration status

   ➤ Fear of medical experimentation or research

   ➤ Fear of allopathic medications or treatment recommendations

   ➤ History of traumatic experiences

      ➤ Posttraumatic stress disorder in patients who have survived civil wars, genocides, ethnic clashes, refugee status, forced migrations

   ➤ Culture-specific health issues

      ➤ Risk factors for certain diseases

      ➤ Systems of culturally based health values, beliefs, and behaviors

      ➤ Variations in response to treatment

➤ *Institutional/practice requirements:*

  ➤ Adequate interpreter services

  ➤ Diverse staff and providers

  ➤ Available translated forms and assessment tools

  ➤ Use of cultural guides/brokers and community leaders

  ➤ Multicultural expertise and representation on ethics committees

  ➤ Awareness of one's own personal biases and implications for practice style

➤ *Health disparities:*

  ➤ Disparities in health *care* vs health *status* (both exist)

    ➤ Health care disparity: concerns the delivery of health care

    ➤ Health status disparity: concerns the health of people in a certain population

  ➤ Documented to exist for multiple factors

    ➤ Mortality rates are worse for ethnic/minority older adults

    ➤ Morbidity may be greater because ethnic/minority elders often present at later and more advanced disease stages

    ➤ Differences in access to health care

    ➤ Utilization of health care services/resources

      ➤ Ethnic elders use formal health care services less than majority population

        ➤ Primary care and preventive services

        ➤ Health education and counseling

        ➤ Mental health services

        ➤ Formal long-term care services

      ➤ Some services are used more frequently by elderly patients

        ➤ Emergency department

        ➤ Acute care

    ➤ Quality of care

    ➤ Performance of procedures, diagnostic testing, preventive measures

➤ *Why disparities exist for ethnic/minority elders:*

  ➤ Language discordance

  ➤ Low health literacy levels

  ➤ Financial factors

    ➤ Lack of insurance coverage

      ➤ Older adults who have not worked and/or paid taxes in the United States for enough time are not eligible for Social Security or Medicare

    ➤ Poverty is linked to poorer self-reported health status, and more older minority adults meet federal poverty criteria than mainstream population

    ➤ Immigration status

  ➤ Poor access to care

    ➤ Services unavailable in community

    ➤ Lack of knowledge about services

    ➤ Geographic constraints (eg, transportation)

    ➤ Physical environment

      ➤ Patient's living situation

      ➤ Ability to navigate health care settings

  ➤ Most disparities are most pronounced for the groups that are growing the fastest

  ➤ Genetic/biological factors

  ➤ Socioeconomic status

  ➤ Personal/cultural beliefs and attitudes toward allopathic/ Western medicine

  ➤ Alienation from/distrust of medical system based on past personal or historical experiences of minorities

➤ *Complementary and alternative/traditional medicine:*

  ➤ Respect culturally decided choices such as consulting or using folk healers, spiritual guides

➤ *Use of language interpreters:*

  ➤ Resources available

  ➤ Guidelines for appropriate use (refer to Table 32-1)

➤ Have presession meetings to discuss roles and expectations.

➤ Speak in short units.

➤ Minimize use of technical terminology, slang, jargon, metaphors, and idioms.

➤ *Face the patient and address him/her directly*, not the interpreter.

  ➤ Patients with hearing impairment may have difficulty hearing the telephone interpreters; if using an in-person interpreter, ensure that the patient can see the interpreter's mouth and gestures

➤ Be patient.

➤ Do *not* use children or other family members as interpreters.

➤ *Use of standardized assessment instruments:*

  ➤ Must assess patient's language literacy and fluency

  ➤ Ensure appropriateness for patient's educational level

  ➤ Be aware of established population norms

  ➤ Be aware of sensitive issues

    ➤ Depression, anxiety, psychiatric/psychological issues

    ➤ Cognitive impairments, dementias

    ➤ Functional status assessments

    ➤ Informed consent (eg, addressing potential negative outcomes/alternatives)

    ➤ Advance care directives

➤ *Community involvement:*

  ➤ Getting to know local community increases your visibility, acceptance, and accountability

  ➤ Also shown to decrease health disparities

    ➤ Conducting a community needs assessment

      ➤ Review local/state census health data

      ➤ Review patient medical records (can be a quality assurance project)

      ➤ Collect data from patients on their needs

        ➤ Focus groups/surveys

        ➤ Patient satisfaction assessments before and after interventions

➤ *Collaborate with local community leaders:*

  ➤ Cultural brokers and community health ambassadors

  ➤ "Promotores de salud"

    ➤ Community health workers

    ➤ Serve as bridge between community members and health care services

  ➤ Cultural, religious, and senior centers

  ➤ Social service agencies

  ➤ Aldermen and other locally elected political representatives

➤ *Monitoring conditions with known disparities in your practice:*

  ➤ Process of care

    ➤ Monitoring, testing, referral patterns, prescribing patterns

    ➤ Review of convenience of hours, staff diversity, disparity training, signage, and written educational materials

  ➤ Patient satisfaction

  ➤ Outcomes of care

  ➤ Can be a quality assurance project

CHALLENGES

➤ Lack of self-awareness on physicians' part

➤ Time constraints

➤ Financial issues

➤ Language

➤ Inadequate knowledge/biased beliefs about patient populations

SOLUTIONS

➤ Staff/provider training

  ➤ Can use a variety of faculty/staff development modules available on the Web (see below)

- ➤ Download information from various sites to create your own curriculum

- ➤ Use materials in the Useful Resources section at the end of this chapter

- ➤ Implicit Association Test

  - ➤ https://implicit.harvard.edu/implicit/

  - ➤ Provides insight into providers' own biases and allows for further exploration combined with specific exercises (see Box 32-1)

- ➤ Tools to help assess and communicate in cross-cultural settings

  - ➤ The LEARN Mnemonic[8]

    - ➤ Providers **Listen** with sympathy and understanding

    - ➤ Patient **Explains** his or her perceptions of the problem

    - ➤ **Acknowledge** differences

Box 32-1 Questions for Addressing Cultural Self-Awareness

1. How do you define your own racial or ethnic identity?

2. What did you learn to value while you were growing up?

3. What are some of the features of your own racial or ethnic group that you view positively?

4. What are some of the features of your own racial or ethnic group that you view negatively?

5. While you were growing up, were the schools and neighborhoods homogeneous or racially and/or ethnically mixed? At what point in your life did you have the opportunity to interact with people who were different from you?

6. Are there other racial or ethnic groups with which you feel comfortable?

7. Are there other racial or ethnic groups with which you feel uncomfortable?

8. What is the racial/ethnic or sociocultural characteristic of patients with whom you feel most competent in establishing rapport and establishing a treatment plan?

9. What is the racial/ethnic or sociocultural characteristic of patients with whom you have the most difficulty establishing rapport and establishing a treatment plan?

10. How do factors related to your racial or ethnic identity and/or from your life experience affect how you interact with patients from backgrounds that are different from your own?

Adapted from Goldman R, Monroe AD, Dube C. Cultural self-awareness: a component of culturally responsive patient care. *Ann Behav Sci Med Educ.* 1996;3:37–46.

- **Recommend** treatment
- **Negotiate** to agreement

- The Kleinman Questions/Explanatory Models of Illness[9]

  - *What do you call your illness? What name does it have?*

  - *What do you think has caused the illness?*

  - *Why and when did it start?*

  - *What do you think the illness does? How does it work?*

  - *How severe is it? Will it have a short or long course?*

  - [For the provider to ask him/herself] *What kind of treatment do you think the patient should receive? What are the most important results you hope he or she receives from this treatment?*

  - *What are the chief problems the illness has caused?*

  - *What do you fear most about the illness?*

  - *What kind of treatment would you like to have? What are the most important results you hope to get from treatment?*

- The ETHNIC Model to improve cross-cultural communication[10]

  - Patient's **Explanation** of symptoms

  - Remedies/medicines tried by patient in **Treating** the illness

  - Has patient sought the help of **Healers**?

  - **Negotiation** of options that are mutually acceptable

  - **Interventions** that include patient's preferences

  - **Collaboration** with family, friends, community members/leaders, interdisciplinary team

TAKE-HOME POINTS

- *Every* patient encounter represents a cross-cultural encounter.

- Diversity of the aging population is increasing.

- All providers need to be prepared to handle issues in cross-cultural care.

➤ There is a need to target interventions to reduce health disparities.

➤ Web sites and publications are readily available for the busy practitioner.

USEFUL RESOURCES

Resources for Using Medical Interpreters, Linguistic Issues

➤ Diversity Rx.

  ➤ (www.diversityrx.org/).

  ➤ Clearinghouse of information on how to meet the language and cultural needs of minorities, immigrants, refugees, and other diverse populations seeking health care.

  ➤ Impact of language/culture on health care.

  ➤ Model programs, best practices, training courses, quality assessments.

  ➤ Laws and regulations regarding equal access to health care services.

  ➤ Role of linguistically and culturally appropriate services in assuring quality, improving cost-effectiveness, and responding to managed care regulations and accreditation guidelines.

➤ Robert Wood Johnson Foundation: Hablamos Juntos.

  ➤ (www.hablamosjuntos.org/default.asp).

  ➤ Addresses language needs for the rapidly growing Spanish-speaking population.

➤ California Endowment.

  ➤ (www.calendow.org/uploadedFiles/language_access_issues.pdf).

  ➤ Toolkit for addressing language issues in your office/practice.

  ➤ Includes information/training modules for office staff and providers.

➤ Translating tools.

  ➤ Multiple free sites available online.

  ➤ Need to be careful of literal translating, limitations with medical terminology, and literacy level of patient/family.

➤ Translated assessment tools (see Table 32-2).

Resources Providing Information on Ethnicity and Aging, Curricula for Teaching/Training

➤ Ethnomed.

  ➤ (http://ethnomed.org/).

  ➤ Information about cultural beliefs, medical issues, and related topics pertinent to the health care of immigrant.

➤ National Center for Cultural Competence.

  ➤ (www11.georgetown.edu/research/gucchd/nccc/index.html).

  ➤ Training, tools, resources for various aspects of cross-cultural care.

TABLE 32-2 Translated Standardized Assessment Tools

Measurement Domain	Standardized Assessment Instruments (English)	Additional Languages
Cognitive	Blessed Dementia Rating Scale	Spanish
	Boston Naming Test	Spanish
	Comprehensive Assessment and Referral Interview	Spanish
	Cognitive Abilities Screening Instrument	Chinese, Japanese, Spanish, Vietnamese
	Geriatric Mental State	Chinese, Spanish
	ICD-9/10 (International Classification of Diseases)	Chinese, Italian, Japanese, Korean
	Iowa Screening Test	Romanian, Russian, Yiddish
	IQCODE: Informant Questionnaire on Cognitive Decline in the Elderly	French
	Kahn-Goldfarb Mental Status Questionnaire (MSQ)	Spanish
	MMSE: Mini-Mental State Examination	Chilean, Chinese, German, Greek, French, Maltese, Russian, Spanish, Thai
	NINCDS-ADRDA: National Institute of Neurological and Communicative Disorders and Stroke and the Alzheimer's Disease and Related Disorders Association	French, Italian, Nigerian, Spanish
	SPMSQ: Short Portable Mental Status Questionnaire	Spanish
	WAIS: Wechsler Adult Intelligence Scale R	Spanish
Emotion	CES-D: Center for Epidemiological Studies–Depression	Chinese, Japanese, Korean, Spanish, Filipino
	Depression Adjective Checklist	Chinese, Hebrew, Spanish, Vietnamese
	DSM: Diagnostic and Statistical Manual of Mental Disorders	Chilean, Chinese, German, Lebanese, French, Italian, Japanese, Korean, Spanish
	Geriatric Depression Scale (GDS)	Chinese, Korean, Spanish
	Hamilton Depression Scale	German, Greek, Russian
	MMPI: Minnesota Multiphasic Personality Inventory	Japanese, Korean, Spanish

(continued)

TABLE 32-2 *(continued)*

Measurement Domain	Standardized Assessment Instruments (English)	Additional Languages
	OARS: Old Americans Resources and Services	Japanese, Korean
	Self-rating Depression Scale	Japanese, Spanish
	State-Trait Anxiety Scale	More than 40 languages
Function	DAFS: Direct Assessment of Functional Status	Spanish
	International Activities of Daily Living (ADL) Scale	German, Greek, Russian
	Katz ADL	Spanish

➤ Stanford Geriatric Education Center: Ethnogeriatrics.

　➤ (http://sgec.stanford.edu/).

　➤ Ethnogeriatrics curriculum, information about different ethnic elder groups in the United States.

　➤ Opportunities for faculty training/development.

　➤ Webinars on various topics in ethnicity and aging.

　➤ Books and other resources.

➤ Doorway Thoughts: cross-cultural health care for older adults.

　➤ http://www.americangeriatrics.org/publications/shop_publications/education__clinical_tools_for_health_care_providers/

　➤ Series of three books published by the American Geriatrics Society.

　➤ Also available as a fan-deck for quick reference.

　➤ Addresses practical issues for practitioners.

　　➤ Caring for older adults from different ethnic/minority groups.

　　➤ Caring for older adults from different religious backgrounds.

　　➤ Case-based studies and questions highlighting key issues.

Resources for Population Statistics

➤ Agency for Healthcare Research and Quality (AHRQ).

　➤ Numerous databases addressing health disparities, health status.

　➤ (www.ahrq.gov/research/minorix.htm).

　➤ (www.ahrq.gov/research/elderix.htm).

➤ The Office of Minority Health (OMH) and National Standards on Culturally and Linguistically Appropriate Services (CLAS).

    ➤ Data and statistics by ethnic/racial group, health topics.

        ➤ (http://minorityhealth.hhs.gov/templates/browse.aspx?lvl=2&lvlID=15).

    ➤ Training modules in cultural competence, funding opportunities.

        ➤ (http://minorityhealth.hhs.gov/).

➤ US Census Bureau.

    ➤ (www.census.gov/).

    ➤ Wide array of demographic information.

➤ Kaiser Family Foundation.

    ➤ (www.statehealthfacts.org/).

    ➤ Free, up-to-date, and easy-to-use health data on all 50 states.

    ➤ Data on more than 500 health topics including health status, insurance coverage, mortality, access to health care services, minority health.

➤ DiversityData.org.

    ➤ (http://diversitydata.sph.harvard.edu/).

    ➤ Identifies metropolitan area indicators of diversity, opportunity, quality of life, and health for various racial and ethnic population groups.

➤ National Center for Health Statistics (CDC).

    ➤ (www.cdc.gov/nchs/fastats/).

    ➤ (www.cdc.gov/nchs/fastats/map_page.htm).

    ➤ Information on a variety of health care topics nationally and at the state level.

REFERENCES

1. Adelman RD, Greene MG, Ory MG. Communication between older patients and their physicians. *Clin Geriatr Med.* 2000;16(1):1–24.

2. Xakellis G, Brangman SA, Hinton WL, et al. Curricular framework: core competencies in multicultural geriatric care. *J Am Geriatr Soc.* 2004;52:137–142.

3. Adler RA, Kamel HK, Brangman SA, Pan CX, Yeo G, Grudzen M, eds. *Doorway Thoughts: Cross-Cultural Health Care for Older Adults.* Vol 1–3. Sudbury, MA: Jones and Bartlett Publishers; 2004, 2006, 2008.

4. Bigby J, ed. *Cross-Cultural Medicine.* Philadelphia, PA: American College of Physicians; 2003.

5. Curriculum in Ethnogeriatrics, Stanford University Geriatric Education Center. www.stanford.edu/group/ethnoger/. Accessed November 30, 2009.

6. Betancourt JR. *Improving Quality and Achieving Equity: The Role of Cultural Competence in Reducing Racial and Ethnic Disparities in Health Care*. New York, NY: The Commonwealth Fund; October 2006.

7. Flores G. The impact of medical interpreter services on the quality of health care: a systematic review. Med Care Res Rev. 2005 June; 62(3):255–99.

8. Berlin EA, Fowkes WC. A teaching framework for cross-cultural health care: application in family practice.*West J Med*. 1983;139:934–8.

9. Kleinman, A. *Patients and Healers in the Context of Culture*. Berkeley, CA: University of California Press: 1980.

10. Kobylarz FA, Heath JM, Like RC. The ETHNIC(S) mnemonic: A clinical tool for ethnogeriatric education. J Am Geriatr Soc 2002; 50 (9): 1582–1589.